THE ETHICAL FOOD MANIFESTO

CHANGING AMERICA ONE SHOPPING CART AT A TIME

Susie L. Hoeller

July 15, 2009
Dear Frank,
Best wishes!
Susie

Copyright © 2009 Susie L. Hoeller

ISBN 978-1-60145-784-4

All rights reserved. No part of this publication may be reproduced, stored in a retrieval system, or transmitted in any form or by any means, electronic, mechanical, recording or otherwise, without the prior written permission of the author.

Printed in the United States of America.

BookLocker.com, Inc.
2009

DEDICATION

In memory of my late brother, James C. Yovic, a graduate of Hebron Academy in Hebron, Maine and the University of South Florida in Tampa who passed away at age 32 from complications of Type 1 diabetes.

In honor of my brother, William C. Yovic, an economics graduate of Colby College in Waterville, Maine, whose thirty year career in the pharmaceutical and medical device industry has been conducted with the highest integrity.

TABLE OF CONTENTS

Introduction 1

Chapter One: Harmful Effects of Current American Food Policy and Practices 5

Chapter Two: Ethical Standards Applied to Food Policy and Practices in America 18

Chapter Three: Becoming an Ethical Food Consumer 27

Chapter Four: Demanding Transparency in the Food Industry 38

Chapter Five: Reforming Federal Regulation of Food Policy 57

Conclusion 63

Exhibits 67

   Exhibit A: The Peanut Corporation of America 69

   Exhibit B: Pending Reform 82

   Exhibit C: School Lunches 97

   Exhibit D: Bisphenol A 107

   Exhibit E: Supplements 122

Acknowledgements 145

Appendix I: For Further Reading 147

End Notes 151

Introduction

Americans know that something has gone terribly wrong with our nation's food supply. It once was universally regarded as the safest in the world. Today, consumer surveys reveal that our collective trust in food companies has plummeted. This is because we have experienced never ending outbreaks of food poisoning. Recalls of products sold on every aisle of our grocery stores are constantly in the news. Spinach, pet food, peanut butter, baby food, chili, ground beef, peanut containing products, and pistachios are recent examples of national (and international) recalls conducted by food processors and grocery stores. Restaurant chains have been impacted by outbreaks of food poisoning and recalls linked to green onions, lettuce, jalapeño peppers, ground beef, and other menu items.

We have watched food industry executives take the 5th Amendment before televised Congressional hearings and refuse to testify about allegations that they knowingly shipped contaminated peanut products. There are news reports of downer cows, child labor and immigration raids at meat packing plants. Food prices go up while quality and safety go down. More and more Americans are overweight or obese and suffering from Type 2 diabetes and other diet related illnesses. Some companies market unhealthy food as "natural." Children are still served non-nutritious food at many schools and consequently cannot concentrate and learn. In the meantime, 35 million Americans go hungry. Irreplaceable farmland is destroyed for subdivisions and shopping centers, many of them foreclosed on and empty since the Wall Street collapse of last fall.

At the time of this writing in April 2009, Congress is working on new legislation to fix our broken food safety system. However, critics are warning that the proposed legislation will put small farmers and farmers' markets out of business. The concern is that only large scale agribusiness can comply with the new mandates leading to further industrialization of our food supply. Our federal agricultural policies have long favored industrial food production. The negative impacts on small producers, consumer health, animal welfare, and our environment have been largely ignored.

THE ETHICAL FOOD MANIFESTO

In the past few years, many authors have written about the numerous problems in our food industry and have suggested needed reforms. Some of the prominent books are listed in Appendix I to this Manifesto. Rather than re-examine in great detail all of these issues, this book speaks directly to the root cause not just the symptoms.

In my opinion, the most significant root cause of the deficiencies of our food policies is the average American consumer's insatiable demand for large portions of inexpensive food. Politically, it is easier to blame the insufficiently funded Food and Drug Administration (FDA) and the food industry for all of our problems. Congress can pass stricter food safety laws. Multi-national food companies can reformulate their products to make them healthier and limit their advertising to children. However, until the majority of Americans change their shopping, eating and investing habits, thus driving the food industry to respond, any reforms will be marginal at best.

The Ethical Food Manifesto will motivate and empower readers to help change America one shopping cart at a time. President Obama said during his campaign and in his Inaugural Address, that government alone cannot change our country – every American has to be involved and take on personal responsibility. ("For as much as government can and must do, it is ultimately the faith and determination of the American people upon which this nation relies.") If we all start applying ethical principles to our food choices, we will see many personal and societal benefits. Before we identify ethical standards, let us review some of the problems needing to be solved.

Chapter One

Harmful Effects of Current American Food Policy and Practices

American agri-business has successfully produced and distributed an incredible abundance of inexpensive foodstuffs to millions of Americans. Visits to our grocery stores inspire awe in people from poor countries. They cannot believe their eyes when they see the quantity and variety of foodstuffs on our shelves. Food in America is sold at lower retail prices and spending on food represents a much lower percentage of family income as compared with other countries. Here are some revealing statistics from a recent United States Department of Agriculture (USDA) publication:

> The average U.S. consumer spent 9.8% of disposable income on food in 2007;
>
> From 1970-2005, the percentage of disposable income spent on food by Americans as a whole fell from 13.9% to 9.8%;

Prices for food rose 4.0% in 2007 and 2.4% in 2006, one of history's fastest growth periods, but were outpaced by a greater rise in personal income during the same period, 5.7% and 5.9% respectively;

Lower income consumers spend a much larger portion of their income on food, up to 25% of their disposable income.[1]

While industrialized nations generally devote a smaller fraction of personal income to food than less developed countries, Americans spend the least by far. The average American spends 5.7% of income annually on food to be prepared at home, much less than other industrialized powers such as the United Kingdom (8.6%) or Germany (11.4%). Other modern countries, like France, Japan, and South Korea, spend more than double what Americans spend. Some economically powerful nations (Mexico at 24.2%, China at 34.9%, and Russia at 28.9%) spend an even larger proportion, and developing nations (Pakistan and Indonesia at 45.7%) commonly spend close to half of disposable income on food.[2] American priorities and values have become confused when we, as consumers, are more willing to devote vast sums of money toward luxury items than on ensuring the safety of the food we eat.

Despite all of this abundance, thirty-five million Americans do not have enough nutritious food to eat. The Bush Administration callously labeled these Americans as suffering from "food insecurity." Hunger and malnutrition are the more accurate descriptions of their situation. The "Food Stamp Challenge," in which civic leaders and ordinary citizens commit to living on a food stamp budget for a period of time, is bringing greater public attention to the hunger problem. A civic leader in my community recently participated in the Food Stamp Challenge where she could only spend $25 a week on food. She came from a family where worrying about grocery bills was never an issue. Living on the food stamp budget, she became light headed and had difficulty concentrating at work. Instead of going down the aisles in the grocery store and putting whatever she wanted in her cart, she had to plan very carefully. She could not afford the meat and chicken she was accustomed to eating. The program helped her realize that many parents go hungry so their children have enough to eat. She is now working with our local food bank and spreading the word about her life changing experience on blogs and Twitter. Like other dedicated citizens, this leader is working to change the status quo and help provide nutritious food for Americans who have been laid off from their jobs or otherwise are in need.

For the vast majority of Americans, the problem has not been too little food but too much food. Our rates of obesity and related illnesses have skyrocketed in recent years. In the United States, almost 25 million children are obese or overweight. The current generation of American children could be the first to have shorter life spans than their parents.

There are organizations fighting to reverse these trends. Former President Bill Clinton has worked tirelessly to combat the serious problem of childhood obesity through The Alliance for a Healthier Generation, a partnership between the Clinton Foundation and the American Heart Association. With its Healthy Schools Program, the Alliance has helped schools adopt healthier lunch menus, replace soft drinks in school vending machines, involve children in more exercise, and teach them healthy eating habits.

The Council of Better Business Bureaus (BBB) has established the Children's Food and Beverage Advertising Initiative. Participating companies pledge to refrain from using advertising directed to children under 12 for products that fail to meet nutritional guidelines approved by the BBB. The purpose of this program is to encourage children to make healthy diet choices and exercise more.[3]

Former Arkansas Governor and 2008 Republican presidential candidate, Mike Huckabee has written about his successful battle against obesity in his book, *Quit Digging Your Grave with a Knife and Fork: A 12-Step Program to End Bad Eating Habits and Begin a Healthy Lifestyle.*

The Obama Administration has been in office less than 100 days. First Lady Michelle Obama has already drawn Americans' attention to our collective need for nutritious, locally grown and accessible food. Mrs. Obama has planted a White House vegetable garden and served healthy meals at shelters in Washington D.C.

Besides obesity, hunger, and the lack of fresh food in inner cities and isolated rural areas, there are many other harmful effects from our current food policy and practices. Much has been written (and revealed on undercover videos filmed by animal protection groups) since the days of Upton Sinclair's classic 1906 expose of the Chicago stockyards in *The Jungle*. The cruel confinement and treatment of livestock and poultry in many factory farms, dairies, feedlots, transport, and processing plants is terrible. However, there are food companies which are leading the way in developing programs to protect the welfare of animals raised for food. McDonald's has implemented and enforced a rigorous system of auditing its supply chain, making it a food industry leader in animal welfare policy. On March 29, 2009, Cargill Meat Solutions announced that it would install a third-party, 24/7 video auditing program at all of its United States slaughter facilities by the end of the year. This program, along with the company's humane animal-handling training and certification programs for employees, should (as the McDonald's program has already done) raise performance standards for the entire meat industry.

Unfortunately, unlike McDonald's and Cargill, there are other meat and poultry companies which mount political and lobbying campaigns to discredit people they view as "aggressive animal rights activists." They do not enforce animal welfare practices on themselves or their suppliers. It is more profitable to raise and slaughter animals and poultry without the added expense of instituting humane facilities and processes. If companies in the American meat and poultry industry had never adopted inhumane and cruel practices to begin with, animal welfare activists could have left them alone and instead focused their energy on other serious issues like ending the disgraceful Canadian seal hunt and protecting whales from Japanese consumers. It is fair to say that most Americans are not opposed to eating animal protein but do want animals and poultry raised for food to be treated humanely. After all, Californians recently passed by nearly a 2-to-1 majority, a ballot initiative that will ban the continued use of cruel pens and cages where pregnant hogs, calves and hens have been unable to stretch out or turn around.

Many farm workers are paid very low wages and work in harsh conditions. Illegal child labor practices were taking place in a kosher meat packing plant in Pottsville, Iowa last year. Where were the USDA inspectors, the rabbis, and the Iowa Department of Agriculture? Where were the business customers of the plant? The plant's numerous violations of child labor, animal welfare and sanitary laws were only discovered when Immigration and Customs Enforcement raided the plant to arrest undocumented immigrant workers.

The overcrowding of livestock and poultry in many agri-business facilities has led to the widespread use of antibiotics. These drugs are needed to keep the animals and fowl alive in unhealthy conditions before slaughter. Antibiotics have entered into our rivers and streams and into our bodies as a result of the food we eat. Resistance to antibiotics for curing infections has grown with their excessive use in agriculture.

Pesticides and herbicides have been overused leading to environmental degradation and loss of habitat for birds and wildlife. Cancer clusters occur in agricultural communities where chemicals sprayed for the mass production of crops are absorbed into the body of local inhabitants.

Small farmers are unable to implement better practices and compete because of so called "efficient" agribusiness relentlessly driving down profit margins. Today, farmers only earn 20 cents for every dollar of food they sell into the general supply chain, whereas the same farmer would have received 40 cents in 1950 and 30 cents in 1980. Much of the food dollar is wasted by the industry on excessive marketing and advertising rather than ensuring consistent quality and safety and paying the farmers their fair share.

Grocery and food service workers in many companies are underpaid and have no affordable health or retirement benefits. They cannot support a family in decent living conditions and form what many commentators describe as the "working poor." Why do Americans continue to accept this state of affairs? If people work full time they should not be poor. It is not ethical to pay workers wages that do not afford a decent living, and this practice should be illegal. Corners have been cut in food processing plants, such as the plants operated by the Peanut Corporation of America. The resulting unsanitary conditions cause outbreaks of food poisoning deaths and illnesses and necessitate the recall of millions of products.

Americans love their "popcorn shrimp" and other imported farm-raised fish, which require destructive aquaculture practices to produce. Worldwide destruction of mangrove forests has been caused by this intensive aquaculture in third world countries. The unregulated use of high levels of chemicals and antibiotics needed to keep the shrimp and fish alive in overcrowded ponds pose health risks to workers. The oceans are being over fished with huge species depletions.

The number of migratory songbirds returning to the United States and Canada has sharply declined due to the use of highly toxic pesticides and chemicals across Latin America during the process of large scale farming for export. "Ornithologists blame the demand for out-of-season fruit and vegetables and other crops in North America and Europe for the destruction of...half of the songbirds that warbled across America's skies only 40 years ago, wiped out by pesticides used south of our border or loss of habitat" for export-led agriculture. "Testing by individual EU countries and the US [FDA] reveals that fruits and vegetables imported from Latin America are three and sometimes four times as likely to violate basic standards for pesticide residues."[4]

Ingredients in every day processed foods like children's cereals flow in from countries with inadequate or non-existent food safety regimes, but the sources of these ingredients are never disclosed to American consumers unless and until a massive national recall occurs. Then, too late, we discover that our pets have died from eating wheat gluten contaminated with melamine added by unscrupulous profiteers overseas.

Some companies take advantage of laxity in the FDA regulations governing health claims and consumer ignorance of processed food ingredients to sell "natural" or "healthy" products that really are neither.

A complete and detailed description of all of these harmful effects and more would take thousands of pages. Readers who desire to know more details can consult some of the books listed in Appendix I or perform their own internet searches. Just type into a search engine words like "food safety," "recall," "downer cows," "child labor," "salmonella," "E-coli," "high fructose corn syrup," "mangrove destruction," and "FDA Import Alerts." Thousands of hits will come up. An excellent source of very current information is a blog published by Dr. Douglas Powell, an associate professor of food safety at Kansas State University (barfblog.foodsafety.ksu.edu).

What can be done to cure these problems? In the near future, thanks to the leadership of Rosa DeLauro (D-CT) and Henry Waxman (D-CA) in the House of Representatives, and Senators Dick Durbin (D-IL) and Lamar Alexander (R-TN), Congress will soon pass new food safety legislation. The FDA will finally be granted mandatory recall authority. There will be increased funding for FDA inspections of U.S. food processing plants and imported foods. Perhaps the food safety programs of the FDA and the USDA will be combined into a single agency. There will be new, government imposed, supply chain traceability requirements. But only large companies will have the financial and human resources to comply with many of the current proposals and implementation of new regulations will not completely cure all of our problems. More funding and legal powers for the FDA and USDA are needed but this alone will not address the underlying root cause of our broken system – which is the demand of so many American consumers for huge portions of inexpensive and often unhealthy food - no matter the "collateral damage."

Chapter Two

Ethical Standards Applied to Food Policy and Practices in America

Ethical conduct is generally described as making choices between right and wrong. The ethical person will freely choose right conduct over wrong conduct. In most societies, historically and today, the murder of another human being is a crime. However, Americans have had difficulty in agreeing on a consistent ethic around what types of killing constitute murder. Clearly, an armed robber who shoots and kills a defenseless convenience store clerk is universally seen as a murderer and will be punished under our criminal laws. But what about our bombing runs over Iraq and Afghanistan where innocent civilians are killed not only terrorists? Is this murder or just a case of unintended "collateral damage"? The doctor who aborts a 16 week old fetus – is she a murderer of a tiny human being waiting to be born or simply a medical professional terminating a pregnancy?

These two questions show that although ethics involves choosing between right and wrong, there is not always a consensus on what conduct constitutes right or wrong in specific circumstances. Students learn about numerous ethical philosophies and principles, usually named after the originating philosopher or religion upon which the system's ethical norms are based. Some college ethics courses only cover the sources of Western philosophy and religion, while others provide a global perspective.

Professionals are bound by the ethical rules or canons of their profession, such as, legal ethics, medical ethics or accounting ethics. These are instances of "applied ethics" where rules of conduct are tailored to a narrow field. The professionals may memorize the canons like the attorney-client confidentiality rule but never study their philosophical or moral foundations.

Since this Manifesto is not a survey of the world's ethical systems, we will only touch on a few notable philosophers, teachers and religious leaders who have influenced our modern U.S. culture[5] and identify which ethical standards the Manifesto applies.

Ancient Greeks

The ancient Greek philosophers provided an early foundation for Western ethical culture. Plato, a proponent of "ethical egoism," claimed that "the moral life is the life that is the most to our ultimate advantage." His student, Socrates focused on ethical self-reflection, writing that "the unexamined life is not worth living." Aristotle, the founder of "virtue ethics," found a path to virtue through "personal excellence" which then contributes to the good life for society as a whole.

Old Testament Hebrews

The Hebrews saw ethics as springing from the divine command of Yahweh, the exclusive and all powerful Creator. Following God's commandments would lead to right conduct pleasing to God. He would bless his chosen people, the Hebrew tribes of Israel, for their righteous conduct. Interestingly, many of the Old Testament commands deal with proper food sources, food preparation and food service. The Old Testament chronicles the numerous divine punishments and disasters which befell the Hebrews when they ignored God's commands.

Jesus Christ

In the New Testament, Jesus Christ teaches revolutionary ethical ideas to His followers. Rather than a rule based set of divine prohibitions, Jesus called his disciples to practice *agape* love towards others, especially the poor and the marginalized people in Israel; lepers, prostitutes and tax collectors. *Agape* derives from the Greek and can best be described as unselfish love towards others. In fact, Christ's ethical teaching is clearly summarized in one of his most famous sayings: "love your neighbor as yourself." Jesus told his disciples the parable of the Good Samaritan who took care of the traveler he found beaten by thieves and lying alongside the road. This story provides us with a perfect example of applied Christian ethical conduct.

18th Century English Philosophers

In England, at the time of the Industrial Revolution, philosophers such as Jeremy Bentham, John

Stuart Mill and others developed what became known as the "utilitarian" school of ethics. Bentham believed that man's true ethical conduct was governed by his need to avoid pain and seek pleasure. Therefore, the religious concepts of right and wrong were illusory. John Stuart Mill taught that the most ethical action was one which brought the greatest number of people happiness. This thinking led to the creation of principles that govern the modern Western world: the "cost-benefit" analysis in business; majority rule in a democracy; and the "invisible hand" theory of market economies.

Immanuel Kant

Kant, an 18th century Prussian philosopher, emphasized man's duty to perform a particular action because the action is inherently right and without any calculation about the consequences of the action. Kant's ethical philosophy was to "always treat humanity, whether in you or in other people, as an end in itself and not a mere means."

Ayn Rand

In the mid 20th century, Any Rand and her objectivist philosophy placed rational self interest as the highest form of ethical conduct. According to Rand, "Man—every man—is an end in himself, not the means to the ends of others. He must exist for his own sake, neither sacrificing himself to others nor sacrificing others to himself. The pursuit of his own rational self-interest and of his own happiness is the highest moral purpose of his life."

Carol Gilligan and Nel Noddings

In 1982, Gilligan wrote the highly influential book, *A Different Voice: Psychological Theory and Women's Development*. Her view is that a unique voice is expressed by some women. She describes this unique voice as "care" which emphasizes empathy as contrasted with justice which focuses on abstract principles of fairness and equality.

Like Gilligan, Noddings, the author of *Caring: A Feminine Approach to Ethics and Moral Education* (1984) contends that ethics and morality based only on rules or principles are inadequate. Instead, ethics should capture what is distinctive about female moral thinking - the caring for others, such as, a mother caring for her children as well as the importance women place on nurturing human relationships.

Peter Singer

In *Animal Liberation* (1975), Singer expanded the ethical community beyond human beings to include other moral beings – animals. He upended the conventional attitude that animals are ours to use only for our own purposes and without consideration that they are living and feeling creatures.

Rather than select one philosophy for the ethical analysis of our food policy and practices, this Manifesto takes ideas from Jesus Christ, Kant, Gilligan, Noddings, and Singer. Our food choices should not be based only on saving pennies for ourselves and demanding that industry produce and distribute food in the cheapest way possible, while ignoring many external costs. Rather it should be based on a caring concern for the public health, the people who produce and market our food, the animals, and the environment.

American food policies and practices should no longer be driven by consumers' desires to eat huge portions of cheap food. Many Americans suffer from food addictions and eating disorders. There needs to be better mental and physical health treatments available for people with these addictions and disorders following in the footsteps of successful programs like Alcoholics Anonymous. My writing about the poor eating habits or often gluttonous eating habits of Americans is not meant to be personally disparaging or hurtful to any individual. It is just a fact that millions of Americans are overweight or obese. In many communities, where being overweight is more the norm than the exception, people may not even realize how seriously they are abusing their health with over eating and eating non-nutritious food as their primary diet.

As discussed earlier, Americans spend far less on groceries as a percentage of their incomes than people in other countries because our current food production system only accounts for immediate monetary burdens.

Too many people who live in nice homes, drive expensive cars, and purchase all the latest electronic devices, are constantly complaining about their grocery bills, which constitute the smallest percentage of their monthly spending. To me, their priorities are sadly misplaced.

Chapter Three

Becoming an Ethical Food Consumer

We are what we eat.

The **first step** in becoming an ethical food consumer is becoming more informed about what is really going on in our food industry. This is easy to do with all of the resources on the internet.

The **second step** is adopting relevant ethical principles from Jesus Christ (the Golden Rule); Immanuel Kant (humanity is not a mere means); Carol Gilligan and Nel Noddings (empathy and caring for others); and Peter Singer (animals are moral beings and part of the community).

The **third step** is to apply these ethical principles to our food buying, consuming and investing practices as well as our political participation. This means seeking out nutritious food that was produced in a holistic manner where the workers were not exploited, the animals were not cruelly mistreated, the environment was not recklessly degraded, and food safety was not compromised by corner cutting. This means investing in ethical companies not just those with the highest short term profits. Also, it means providing support for political candidates who will work for positive change.

American consumers and investors can no longer blindly trust large segments of the food industry and permit these companies to continue with business as usual. Many people wonder why the pace of food recalls has rapidly accelerated in the past few years. The major reason is because of advanced communication technologies and genetic fingerprinting of microorganisms that cause food borne illness. Today, when people get sick from a food borne illness around the country, the CDC, the FDA, and the state health departments have the technology to track where the illnesses are occurring. The food industry has lagged far behind in its ability to trace where the contaminated food was actually distributed. Yet, the food industry has to take increasing legal and financial responsibility when it makes people sick and/or kills them. Today, it can be scientifically proved through genetic fingerprinting and matching of the food and the sick person's bodily fluids that a particular food caused the illness.

The CDC maintains statistics about the people who are sickened, hospitalized and killed by food borne illnesses. The numbers are staggering especially when we know that people who suffer mild incidences of food poisoning may never seek medical attention. There are approximately 5,000 deaths, 325,000 hospitalizations and 76 million cases of food borne illness in the United States each year.

Until recently, food borne illness cases could not be scientifically traced back to the particular foods and food companies which caused the illness. Food companies were not held truly accountable. Unethical companies took advantage of this situation to adopt unsanitary, negligent, and in some cases, criminal business practices.

This is made abundantly clear from the actions of the Peanut Corporation of America ("PCA"). This outbreak and recall has been on-going for months and involves over 3,900 separate products. The recalled products have been sold by the most prestigious and long established national brands, national supermarket chains, even the higher priced "organic and natural" chains, lesser known private labels, and food service establishments. They have even included Meals Ready to Eat (MREs) for our troops, school lunches, and peanut butter served in nursing homes. The national and private label brands involved in the recall were not exercising sufficient oversight of their peanut ingredient supplier, PCA. If they had, they would not have purchased contaminated peanuts, peanut butter or peanut paste produced in filthy, vermin infested plants in Georgia and Texas. The conditions at PCA are described in more detail in Exhibit A of this book. All of the recalled products are listed on the FDA's website.

At least one major company, Nestle, having properly audited the PCA plant in Texas in 2006, rejected PCA as a supplier based on the results of the their examination of the facility. At a Congressional subcommittee hearing conducted on March 18, 2009, other food companies which purchased peanut butter and peanut products from PCA were asked why they failed to properly audit PCA's facilities and reject PCA as a supplier. Companies selling peanut butter filled crackers and other products, under their own brand names, were criticized by Congressman Bart Stupak (D-MI) for trying to shift the entire blame for salmonella deaths and illnesses to PCA instead of acknowledging their own responsibility to assure the safety of ingredients used in their products.[6]

There are excellent food companies but consumers need to demand a much higher level of transparency from the food industry as a whole for products sold in grocery stores and served in restaurants. The excellent companies have a true commitment to ethical and safe practices, but their identity can be very hard for consumers to determine for reasons set forth below. If a particular company will not improve its practices, then consumers need to stop purchasing from it and only reward companies that consistently adhere to ethical practices in all areas of their business. This is where our shopping carts come in. Yes, we can change America one shopping cart at a time.

We can also contact food companies via email, telephone and postal mail to express our concerns. When companies start hearing from more concerned consumers, this will motivate them to change. Too many food companies only offer broad platitudes about their products and their corporate social responsibility but never provide any concrete data to back up their spin. Their websites focus on marketing hype and recipe suggestions. Many companies simply refuse to provide their customers with any substantive information about the country of origin of ingredients, supply chain and production quality assurance, traceability, animal welfare, and food safety programs. Or if there is a description, it is very brief and broad brushed.

In today's food marketing environment, it is very difficult or even impossible to take the second step because most of the food industry practices are simply not transparent enough to allow for informed consumer choices. Here is some anecdotal data to back up this claim. My husband Ted contacted twelve food companies beginning on March 19, 2009. He selected the companies based on products we have in our pantry. He asked the companies eight questions (paraphrased below) either on the telephone or via email or both:

Do you have any imported ingredients in your products?

Why do you not disclose on your website or labels where the various individual ingredients come from?

What is your traceability system?

Do you audit your suppliers directly or use third party auditors?

What are your animal welfare policies and how are they enforced?

What percent of your budget is spent on food safety as compared to marketing?

How can I, as a consumer, trust your brand when over 3,900 separate products were recalled from companies due to the Peanut Corporation of America? It was dog food before that, spinach, tomatoes, ground beef, and on & on. How do I know your brand is safer than the competitors?

Do you have Bisphenol A in your container liners?

Two of the companies surveyed were privately held. One company sells baked beans and the other one sells kosher products. The baked bean firm was contacted by telephone and provided an immediate and detailed response. This company has direct contact with all their growers and does not use wholesale brokers, therefore their traceability is excellent. Their production and food safety processes were verbally described to my husband in great detail. However, the company representative stated that since the company meets FDA requirements, there is no need to provide any of this detail on the product labels or the company website. They do use cans with Bisphenol A liners because the FDA currently allows it. As a privately held company, they did not want to provide any financial information about their spending on food safety versus marketing. Basically, they appeared to be well run, described safe production methods, and were very direct in their answers. It appears that as a smaller company they have the advantage of more immediate contact with the growers.

The privately held kosher food company owner was very courteous when speaking with my husband. He told Ted that it was a very busy season for his business, and promised to get back to him with substantive responses to the questions.

The other ten companies contacted were publicly traded national brands and, except for a major yogurt maker, they were very difficult to deal with. The highly responsive yogurt company promptly sent Ted a detailed email from a senior level manager addressing his questions in a substantive manner.

Three of the other public companies placed Ted on hold for 15 plus minutes and their representatives were unable to answer any of his questions. Therefore, he sent them an email on their "contact us" website menu and provided the eight questions in writing. So far he has not received any replies from these three companies even though over three weeks have passed since his initial contacts.

When he pressed for information from the remaining six companies on the telephone, Ted was transferred back and forth among various departments, such as Consumer Relations, Human Resources, Public Relations, Corporate Communications, Quality Control, Grocery Products Division, Home Office, and World Headquarters. None of these six companies would answer the eight questions except with vague generalities. They essentially stated that since they meet FDA requirements they have no interest in answering specific consumer questions about their quality assurance, supply chain and food safety processes.

Most of the websites, labels and other material Ted reviewed were more concerned with recipes, new products, how great the company is, and pretty product pictures. One company, unwilling to provide any information about what countries its ingredient were sourced from, told Ted that consumers are simply not interested in receiving this type of information. Another company refused to provide any details about their food safety programs because they consider such information to be "proprietary." Why should this information, which directly impacts the health of their customers, be such a closely guarded secret?

Ethical companies should be proud to tell their customers how much they spend on food safety and explain details of their programs instead of hiding behind the "proprietary" excuse. When they get sued for food poisoning, much of this information is disclosed in discovery to individual plaintiffs anyway. However, companies will apply to the judge for a protective order so that the plaintiff has to keep this information confidential.

THE ETHICAL FOOD MANIFESTO

The general public is kept in the dark and is supposed to "trust" the food companies to always do the right thing.

The twelve companies contacted make canned, boxed and packaged items such as: green beans, baked beans, beef tamales, Catalina salad dressing, freestone peaches, microwave popcorn, yogurt, breakfast cereal, beef gravy, potato pancakes, chicken soup, and vegetable soup.

As stated above, only the privately held baked bean company and the publicly traded yogurt company substantively answered some or all of the eight questions in a timely manner. At least the owner of the kosher foods company has promised a reply after his busy season. The nine unresponsive companies display an arrogant lack of respect for their customers.

Chapter Four

Demanding Transparency in the Food Industry

I strongly encourage Congress to include in the final food safety reform legislation a strong provision requiring food companies to become fully transparent in the areas discussed below. Then consumers will finally be able to knowledgeably choose between companies that truly invest sufficient resources in food safety and companies that do not.

After all, in the wake of the global financial system melt down, at the recent G-20 financial summit meeting in London, leaders of the G-20 countries, including President Obama, agreed to institute new transparency requirements for the global financial industry.

In the meantime, without waiting for Congressional action, some innovative companies are beginning to see the advantage of voluntarily providing consumers with access to their supply chains and traceability systems by using the internet. Companies such as Stone-Buhr Flour and Askinosie Chocolate use "Find the Farmer" websites to reconnect farmer and consumer. A farmer's contact information is on product packaging, and consumers can see where and how their food is grown by viewing the farmer's website. These companies realize the market advantage of incurring marginal costs to create a transparent traceability system, as compared with the massive costs, reputational damage, and enormous waste of a product recall.[7]

The most desperately needed change in the food industry is full and honest transparency. Without it consumers and investors cannot make ethical choices. Transparency is different than the self serving spin or platitudes found on company websites. It means going beyond the financial statements required by Securities and Exchange Commission (SEC). These filings currently do not disclose how much companies are investing in food safety, traceability, animal welfare, etc. Calling for more transparency does not mean improperly asking for disclosure of true trade secrets like the Coca Cola® formula or the Kentucky Fried Chicken Original Recipe®.

The space on most food labels is taken up with marketing photos and broad puffing claims. In most cases, the required ingredient listing and nutritional information is in small print, which is legal under the current law, but not always easy for consumers to read. SEC reports provide information on total sales and cost of goods sold, but it is impossible to determine from them what most of the publicly traded companies are specifically investing in food safety and quality assurance. Expenses for advertising and marketing are stated but quality assurance and food safety may be buried under "research and development."

Today, you can go online to the SEC's EDGAR database and look at food company annual and quarterly reports. Do you feel comfortable with the level of disclosure on quality assurance, food safety and supply chain traceability? Do you want to invest in a food company that causes the next national food poisoning outbreak and recall due to poor quality assurance?

By way of illustration, Con Agra and Menu Foods reported direct expenses in excess of $50 million each for their 2007 recalls of peanut butter and pet food. These figures do not include the litigation related expenses and settlements just the costs of actually conducting the recalls. Both companies have worked hard since 2007 to invest more resources in food safety and rebuild their brands but clearly the companies' reputations were damaged by the 2007 high profile recalls. In fact, at the beginning of the Peanut Corporation of America recall in January 2009, Con Agra, J.M. Smucker, and other national brand makers of peanut butter had to run ads telling consumers that their brands were not part of the PCA recall. Nevertheless, peanut butter sales nationwide have taken a nose dive.

The following is a list of the types of information consumers and investors alike should be able to easily access from company websites, SEC reports, and where practicable, on food labeling and marketing literature.

Traceability – This relates to the ability of the manufacturer or food service establishment to know exactly where their ingredients and products were sourced from and to make sure their entire supply chain is practicing food safety and quality assurance. The lack of traceability has cost the industrialized food industry millions and millions of dollars in recalls and has caused many innocent smaller companies to go bankrupt when the source of contamination cannot be readily identified. In the past two years, the Florida tomato growers and the Texas spinach farmers had nothing to do with alleged tomato and actual spinach contaminations that originated in other states and yet their products had to be recalled as a precaution to protect the public. Millions of tons of food are thrown away which may or may not be safe because no one knows where the contamination originated.

    The defense and electronics industries have had excellent traceability systems in place for decades. Radio Frequency Identification (RFID) is one of the technologies that can successfully improve the global food traceability system. Invented by Texas Instruments in 1989, RFID was immediately adopted by pig farmers in Holland to track their livestock as a way to curtail the spread of animal diseases and enhance food safety. American agri-business as a whole has resisted RFID, the incremental costs of which are extremely low, especially when compared to the lost sales and reputational damage in being part of a national recall. Many ranchers oppose any government proposals to require use of RFID to track livestock herds because they philosophically don't like government programs that interfere with their business (except for taxpayer funded agricultural subsidies) and are worried that the information about the size and growth patterns of herds will be misused by meatpackers to lower prices paid for cattle and other animals. This is a valid concern that can be addressed by the USDA oversight if and when its current National Animal Identification System moves from voluntary to compulsory use of RFID.

On March 23, 2009, IBM ran a full page advertisement in *The New York Times* under the banner "A smarter planet needs smarter food." The advertisement starts off with a list of the high profile recalls of peanut butter, milk, baby food, and spinach. It goes on to say "In the U.S. alone, 300 million pounds of meat and poultry products were recalled between 1994 and 2007. ... And consumers increasingly demand to know more about the food they buy; such as how animals were raised ... it is understandable when there are 76 million cases of food-borne illnesses every year in the U.S. alone."

The advertisement then explains in detail how IBM is building a technology infrastructure to potentially track "every chicken breast, every pork chop, every lamb shank and every beef filet they produce for the Norwegian food market" with Matiq, a subsidiary of Norway's largest food supplier.

"The [Matiq] system will enable the packaging of products with RFID tags to help keep them in optimal condition. At the production factory, sensors will be encoded with data and included with each piece of meat. ...the system will provide ... the farm of origin and the animal's age and health records ... Norwegian food suppliers and supermarkets will have more and better information about the meat they sell ... Matiq's smart food system can help suppliers and grocers reduce costs and improve safety. Even more importantly, it can increase consumers' confidence in the quality of food they purchase ...."

American producers can learn much about advanced food traceability systems from our trading partners in Europe, Argentina, Australia, and New Zealand. In the European Union, for example, cattle have passports tracing their movements from birth to slaughter and fruit is labeled with edible ink to show its origin.

The sad irony is that while American technology companies invent innovative solutions that are adopted in other countries, many American food producers not using this technology. Our food companies then fall behind our trading partners as they continue their outmoded business practices –spending millions upon millions of dollars for fancy product labeling and expensive television commercials instead of infrastructure technology systems that protect the health and safety of their customers.

Again, the root cause is that the vast majority of American consumers are simply not demanding rapid change and innovation in the food industry. We used to be the world leaders in so many scientific and technical fields. Yet in recent years, for a variety of reasons, other countries are surpassing us. Americans riled up by extremist talk show hosts are content to blame Wall Street and Congress for all our problems and those two institutions do need reform. However, many of our problems are created by American consumers' self indulgent lifestyles focused on mindless entertainments as opposed to civic responsibilities. Hopefully, this will change with the leadership of President and Mrs. Obama. They are working hard to motivate every American to make positive changes that benefit society as a whole as opposed to the "me first and me only" thinking that has dominated our country in recent years.

Country of Origin**–**Today, consumers buy a box of children's cereal or a frozen dessert and the package says that the product was manufactured or distributed by a company in an American city and state. The consumer is not told that numerous ingredients in the cereal or dessert are sourced from several other countries which may lack proper food safety systems.

The country of origin disclosure legislation for single ingredient products was fiercely resisted for years by the food industry. It is finally being implemented for meat, seafood, fruits, vegetables, and nuts. Multi-ingredient packaged or processed foods and food service establishments still do not have to reveal the countries of origin for their ingredients. The label on a canned, frozen or packaged product which reads "Manufactured by" or

"Distributed by" followed with the name of an American company gives the consumer the false sense of security that all the ingredients in the package came from the U.S. The truth is that with our global food supply chain, many ingredients come from countries with poor to nonexistent food safety regimes because they are cheap.

Co-Packing Disclosure – Many national brands charge more than store brands based on their national brand advertising. Until recalls revealed that products from national brands and store brands were being made at the same plants, on the same production lines, and recalled with the same frequency, I always used to think that all the national brands were worth paying more for because they represented greater quality and safety. I don't think that way anymore because I can look on the FDA website and see the same products recalled by both the national brands and store private label brands.

In the peanut recall, the national brands and the high end grocery stores recalled products along with private label brands and the discount supermarkets. The pistachio recall which started the first week of April 2009 was kicked off when Kraft Foods testing found salmonella contamination in pistachios sourced from a California processing plant. Kraft should be commended for its supply chain testing program but, just as with the still on-going peanut recall, the contaminated pistachios are being sold under multiple brand names all over the country.

One plant can impact thousands of end products all over the country. This shows that food processing in this country has become too dependent on concentrated, single sourcing. After 9/11, the federal government instituted various programs to prevent bio-terrorism. However, we are not being poisoned by bio-terrorists. It is our own food industry, ridden with food safety failures up and down the supply chains, that is poisoning Americans.

In the meantime, far too often Americans are paying more for attractive packaging and marketing hype not for superior quality and safety. Many of the national brands and the store brands have their products "co-packed" by a third party and not manufactured in plants that they own or control. We saw this with the Con Agra peanut butter recall of 2007, where a non-Con Agra plant in Georgia did not pay attention to a leaky roof and windows. This allowed moisture and other unsanitary conditions to contaminate the peanuts Con Agra used to make the peanut butter. Menu Foods which manufactured melamine contaminated pet food for eighty-eight national and store brands was the single source of wet pet food packaged in pouches for all of these brands.

As a consumer, I want to know when I buy a food product whether or not it is being produced by the company that is marketing it or some third party which may or may not be properly supervised. If there is insufficient room on a can or package label for this disclosure, the information could be placed on the company website. Of course, food companies resist this type of disclosure and hide behind the "burka" of "proprietary information."

Animal Welfare Policies – As IBM said in their advertisement quoted above, more Americans want to know how animals raised for food are being treated. Web cams in slaughter houses would probably turn millions more Americans into vegetarians and vegans just because the killing of animals is a gruesome process even if conducted humanely. If there had been web cams in American slaughterhouses, we would not have had to rely on undercover operations by animal protection groups or immigration raids to find out about sadistic treatment of downer cows and the use of child labor. Thanks to the work of animal protection groups, animal scientists like Dr. Temple Grandin, and companies like McDonald's and Cargill, conditions are greatly improving, but the progress is not universal.

Of course, some followers of Peter Singer, such as People for the Ethical Treatment of Animals (PETA) oppose almost every human "use" of animals. PETA is often derided for its more extreme tactics and campaigns. Nevertheless, the organization has been instrumental in informing millions of people about horrific cruelties inflicted on animals by human beings who mistakenly consider themselves to be civilized and good.

Other animal advocates, such as, The Humane Society of the United States take a different approach when it comes to using animals for food by focusing on humane treatment and not absolute prohibition.

This writer believes that it is ethically acceptable to raise animals for food provided they are treated humanely *in all stages* of the growing and slaughtering process. Otherwise, most animals would never be alive at all since livestock and poultry would not be raised in large numbers as pets. Furthermore, it is not clear to me if a 100% vegetarian or vegan diet is truly healthy. Scientific and nutritional controversies exist over this issue.

Worker Wages and Conditions – With some notable exceptions, it is hard to determine from the food companies themselves specific information about what steps they are taking, if any, to assure that workers who are planting and harvesting crops, tending livestock or working in processing plants have decent wages and working conditions.

We now know that the Peanut Corporation of America paid very low wages to its workforce. There is a direct connection between under paid and dispirited work forces and a lack of food safety. For the most part, food companies do not disclose specifics about these practices. Without the long struggle of the United Farm Workers, co-founded by Cesar Chavez and Dolores Huerta in California, and other organizations, conditions would not have improved. Much more needs to be done in this regard. The farm workers who perform the back breaking work needed to put food on our tables still are not receiving their fair share of our food dollars.

It is encouraging that Florida Republican Governor Charlie Crist met on March 25, 2009 with representatives of the Coalition of Immokalee Workers. This group has been calling on tomato growers in Florida to improve wages and working conditions for pickers and to prevent grower practices that have led to seven federal convictions for modern day slavery in the past ten years. Crist, unlike his predecessor Jeb Bush, is the first Florida governor to meet with this group since the 1990s. As reported by Michael Peltier of naplesnews.com, "Crist is the grandson of a Cypriot who, at 14, emigrated alone to the United States and got his first job shining shoes." After the meeting with the farmworkers, Crist told reporters "I am deeply moved by what they had to say and we want to help them as much as we possibly can … I am not a man driven by anger, much, but two things will: injustice and arrogance."[8]

This coalition of Florida tomato workers has already been successful in persuading Taco Bell, Burger King, Subway, and McDonald's to pay more for tomatoes to improve worker wages.[9] It appears they now have a Florida Governor who is sympathetic to their cause.

Quality Assurance and Food Safety Protocols – All food companies, including grocers and restaurants, have quality assurance and food safety protocols of some sort. With a handful of exceptions, the question that cannot be answered is which companies establish the superior protocols and actually invest the necessary financial and human resources to continuously improve and rigorously enforce them.

Again, for the vast majority of companies, details about these protocols are hidden from consumers behind the burka of proprietary information. Another frequent refrain, heard in the food industry, is that "food safety is not a competitive advantage and we all need to work together to enhance it." It is a good thing for food companies to cooperate in industry associations (within the confines of the antitrust laws) to share quality assurance and food safety best practices. However, sometimes this cooperation and sharing of information only includes other industry participants and is not extended to regulators or consumers. Just like the protection of "proprietary information" excuse, the "food safety is not a competitive advantage" mantra has often been used to keep industry practices hidden from public view.

One of the common industry practices, which came to light as part of the on-going Congressional investigation of the Peanut Corporation of America and reporting by *The New York Times*[10], is the requirement that the producers being audited by their upstream customers in the supply chain pay for the audits themselves. The customers ordering the audit do not pay for it. This questionable practice creates a built in conflict of interest for the auditors. Since they are actually being paid by the plant they are auditing and not the plant's customer, there is a temptation to soften the audit to cozy up to plant management. Obviously, the insufficiently detailed audits performed at the request of customers of the Peanut Corporation of America but paid for by PCA did not influence the hundreds of companies buying ingredients originating from PCA to take their business elsewhere.

If the food industry will not voluntarily reform this questionable practice (which presents an inherent conflict of interest) and start to require that upstream customers pay for the audits of their supply chain as part of their cost of doing business, then Congress should include a prohibition of the practice in the food safety legislation currently being worked on.

Here is a much more positive and inspiring development. On March 30, 2009, Organic Valley Family of Farms, the nation's largest organic cooperative, announced the sharing of its quality assurance and food safety protocols with the entire public as part of its Transparency Initiative. The protocols which had previously been only available as requested by customers, producers, distributors, and retailers, are now posted on the cooperative's website at www.organicvalley.coop/our-story/transparency. The twelve protocols which range from Hazard Analysis of Critical Control Points (HACCP) to the Customer Complaints per Unit Program are described in detail on the website. I would challenge our publicly traded and privately held companies to match or exceed the impressive transparency of Organic Valley.

Chapter Five

Reforming Federal Regulation of Food Policy

Exhibit B provides a summary of the major food safety issues and reform bills pending in Congress as of April 5, 2009. There are many positive ideas in these proposals and there are deficiencies, such as the overburdening of small farms and farmers' markets with costly paperwork requirements. Imposing an excessive administrative burden on small farming operations may have no impact on food safety because most of the food safety problems have arisen in the industrial agriculture and food processing sector. Clearly, the federal government needs more resources and enforcement powers to help assure food safety for both domestically produced and imported food.

In the wake of the lead and magnet toy recalls of 2007, Congress passed the Consumer Product Safety Improvement Act (CPSIA). There are many very good provisions in this new law. Increased penalties will deter and punish manufacturers and sellers of dangerous and defective children's products. Legal protection for employee whistleblowers will make it harder for unethical companies to cover up wrongdoing.

Before the passage of the CPSIA in 2008, it was simply too easy for unethical companies to carelessly or knowingly manufacture or sell defectively designed and manufactured products for children because the profits from their sales far exceeded any potential liabilities or penalties for doing so.

However, there are some problems with this law as well. Vague and overly broad definitions of children's products and unrealistically short implementation dates for new bans and limits on lead and phthalates have resulted in mass confusion in the business community. Inventories of pre-existing products that may have posed no safety risk have had to be destroyed. The massive toy recalls of lead painted toys and toys containing dangerous small magnets involved mass produced overseas items but the CPSIA has burdened American small toy and apparel makers, crafters, thrift shops, and children's booksellers with numerous testing and certification requirements that only large companies can reasonably implement. Even when the Consumer Product Safety Commission (CPSC) later "exempted" crafters and others from some of the testing requirements, many retailers still could not accept their goods without taking undue legal risks or conducting more of their own testing. Of course, I am not contending that small companies or home crafters should be able to make and sell dangerous children's products. I am just pointing out valid criticisms of a law which imposes a "one size fits all" regulatory system on small firms and product categories that were not even the source of defective products that have harmed children. One of the absurdities of the CPSIA's overly broad definitions of "children's products" in the context of lead limits, in the product substrate or on its surface, involves children's ATVs and motorbikes.

"Ever see a kid chewing on the air valve of an ATV tires? Licking the battery? Biting handlebars? They all contain lead and that's the kind of effort it would take for it to endanger kids [with lead poisoning], critics of the regulation say."[11]

I hope that Congress will not make the same mistakes with food safety reforms as it did with some aspects of the CPSIA and recognize that new food safety laws need to be carefully tailored to solve the real problems. We don't need more legislation to be rushed through, like the AIG bailout, without Congressmen actually reading the proposals.

One thing Congress, state legislatures and local governments should do is promote the growth of local and sustainable agriculture, farmers' markets, community gardens, and school gardens with new financial, educational and tax incentives. This will help educate children about where food really comes from and healthy eating, create new jobs, provide fresher foodstuffs, and conserve fuel.

In addition to the growing popularity of farmers' markets, as the general public has become more conscious of the benefits of locally grown food, many regional and national retailers are expanding their presence in this market. Retailers sometimes find it difficult to administer purchasing arrangements with dozens of small local farmers rather than large distributors trucking in produce from huge farms. However, consumer demand is forcing producers and retailers to adjust their practices in a beneficial way. Here are three examples. Growers like Dole have contracted with East Coast farmers to grow broccoli and leafy greens they used to ship from the West Coast. Hannaford Brothers, a New England/New York retailer saw a 20 percent increase in its local produce sales in 2008 as customers voted with their shopping carts for keeping farmland, local farmers, and their money in their own local communities. Plus Hannaford customers want to enjoy fresher produce, are concerned about food safety, and believe that knowing food is coming from local sources is important. In July 2008, Wal-Mart became the biggest purchaser in the locally grown food market by announcing that it would purchase $400 million of locally grown produce over the next year.[12]

The Obama Administration has been emphasizing the creation of "green jobs" to help our economy recover from the global financial crisis. Green jobs have been described as jobs in the energy efficiency sector. The definition needs to be expanded to spur the creation of new and better paying jobs in agriculture, animal science, nutrition science, and food production in our local communities. What could be more "green" than local and sustainable farming?

Conclusion

American farmers and ranchers have produced the most abundant food in the world at the most inexpensive prices. Since the onset of World War I, when Herbert Hoover led successful American efforts to feed millions of starving civilians in war torn Europe, until the present, Americans have been the most generous givers of food aid in the world. It is a record to be proud of. In addition to sending food overseas to relieve hunger, companies like Tyson Foods are sending food technologists and supplies to villages in Rwanda. In cooperation with the Millennium Promise, a non-profit organization working to end extreme global poverty, Tyson is teaching Rwandan women to raise chickens and sell their eggs and meat. The company is also developing school meal programs to increase the protein consumption of Rwandan children.

On the other hand, we have allowed the problems discussed above to fester in our own society. We cannot require that food companies be fully transparent and assure decent wages, animal welfare, and food safety when consumers demand such low food prices that many companies have to cut corners somewhere to survive. We, as consumers, must be willing to pay enough for food so that our food production businesses are healthy, sustainable, and are reasonably profitable. We cannot simultaneously demand excessively low costs as consumers and excessively high returns as investors without examining the external costs. Look what happened to Bernie Madoff's clientele who were seduced with unrealistically high investment returns. At the same time, food companies need to redirect their internal resources away from excessive spending on marketing and advertising and allocate more resources to quality assurance, food safety, animal welfare, workers' wages, and overlay all of this with full and honest transparency.

During the last couple of decades, American culture has mistakenly promoted greed and overconsumption at the top (and in the middle) and exploitation of the so called "working poor" at the bottom. This selfishness and unethical behavior has led to our current financial crisis with its rising unemployment, home foreclosures, and often desperate circumstances for the hardest hit communities and individuals.

However, when conspicuous consumption was the lifestyle goal, millions of Americans overworked themselves and did not spend enough time with their children or in community activities. Many families no longer even took the time to prepare and enjoy healthy meals together.

The current financial crisis has led many Americans in a search to rediscover our country's authentic values and establish a proper balance between work, family and community. As the winds of change renew America, let us adopt an ethical mindset to guide our food policies, choices, and all of our life decisions.

Exhibits

The Exhibits that follow are offered for those who are interested in a more in-depth discussion of five of the current issues that illustrate or expand on the issues discussed in this Manifesto.

Exhibit A: The Peanut Corporation of America

The Peanut Corporation of America ("PCA") had been manufacturing peanut butter in its Blakely, Georgia facility since 2006. PCA developed a specialized role in the peanut butter market by providing low cost peanut butter to institutions, such as schools and nursing homes, as well as large scale distributors for inclusion in cookies, crackers and other products. This business model meant that PCA's products had infiltrated the marketplace throughout the country and into Canada, Europe and New Zealand.

PCA's problems began back in 2001 when the company was only roasting and blanching peanuts, rather than manufacturing peanut butter. At that time, an FDA inspection revealed that equipment in use by the company had not been properly maintained in order to prevent pest infestation and other unsanitary conditions.

After PCA began producing peanut butter, the Georgia Department of Agriculture began conducting inspections of the Blakely facility under a contract with the FDA. These contracts are commonly used by the FDA due to the large number of manufacturing facilities in use and the relatively few federal inspectors employed by the agency. Over the last two years, multiple inspections found sanitation violations at the plant that were reported as minor in nature and corrected by the plant's management on-site. In addition, in August of 2008 a Canadian inspection of some peanut products from this facility revealed metal shavings contained in the product. After salmonella illnesses had already begun to be reported, an inspection on October 23, 2008 noted that the plant's equipment was not being properly maintained and mildew was forming on the ceiling of the facility. Within a month of this inspection, the Centers for Disease Control and Prevention in Atlanta (CDC) began monitoring incidences of salmonella in 16 states across the country.

By early December, the FDA and CDC investigation teams began looking into peanut butter at institutional sources as the cause of the outbreak. The investigation led to the King Nut Company in Ohio, which had received peanut butter from PCA. On January 9, 2009, the FDA began an inspection of the Blakely plant and received information that some of the plant's products had tested positive for salmonella. Within the week, PCA had issued a nationwide recall on all its products. The investigation conducted by the FDA discovered unsanitary conditions at the plant, such as cockroaches, leaking roofs and mold. Even more troubling were PCA's internal records, showing that since 2007 there had been 12 positive salmonella tests at the Blakely facility. After each positive, the company had sought to retest the product at another testing facility, and then continued to ship the product without regard for the prior positive test. After the conclusion of the investigation, the recall was broadened to include all of PCA's products manufactured in Blakely since 2007. The federal government launched a criminal investigation into the methods and procedures that had led to the salmonella outbreak. On February 9, 2009, the FBI raided the Blakely facility in order to obtain evidence and internal memoranda.[13]

Stewart Parnell, the President and Owner of the PCA, had held a seat on the federal government advisory board on peanut quality until early February when the outbreak became public. He was subpoenaed to appear before a hearing of the House Energy and Commerce Committee; however, Parnell refused to answer any of the questions invoking Fifth Amendment protection. The hearing did reveal damaging internal communications by Parnell and the company's practice of retesting products that had previously tested positive for salmonella. One e-mail even shows Parnell complaining that retesting the contaminated products was "costing us huge $$$$$".[14]

The salmonella outbreak has claimed nine lives throughout the country, mostly elderly persons in nursing homes, and caused hundreds of confirmed illnesses (although estimates of actual sicknesses range up to 19,000).[15] PCA shut down another production facility in Plainview, Texas, and filed for bankruptcy protection on February 13, 2008 due to the effects of the massive recall. The recall includes over 3,900 products thus far and has impacted every level of the peanut supply chain, which makes it one of the largest in U.S. history. Although PCA's products did not constitute a large share of the market, at about 2.5%, the industry's integrated supply chain and the impact of this recall on consumer trust has caused sales of peanut butter to plummet for all manufacturers nationwide.[16]

Regulatory Reform

There is an urgent need to reform the way in which the federal government regulates the safety of food throughout the country. Presently, a minimum of 15 different federal agencies have some responsibility for ensuring the safety of food in the country. As Rep. Rosa L. DeLauro stated in a recent hearing, "there is no individual today who is responsible for food safety...We have an immediate crisis which requires a real restructuring."[17] Proposed reforms have discussed the best way in which to create accountability in the regulatory structure surrounding food safety. Most of these reforms have discussed either creating a new agency with the sole responsibility to regulate food safety or strengthening the oversight power of an existing agency.

In this instance, the agency responsible for the safety of peanut butter was the FDA; however, this agency has suffered for years from chronic lack of funding and has limited power to enforce the law. The FDA contracts with 42 states to conduct food safety inspections because it lacks the funding to do so itself. The agency's Science Board recently concluded that it could not ensure the safety of our domestic food supply due to the surge in food manufacturers in recent years. State inspections are not uniform and have proven to be inadequate in many instances. In this case, the recent state inspection of the Blakely facility found only minor violations that were to be corrected by plant management. The subsequent federal investigation found generally unsanitary conditions, a leaky roof over the production area, and salmonella traces present on the production line and the floor.[18]

Under the current FDA rules, the agency was required to seek approval of PCA before expanding the recall of products, even after a criminal investigation into their production methods was announced. Although the FDA does have the power to seize a product that is suspected of contamination or ask a federal judge for authority to recall a product without company approval, these decisive steps are rarely taken by the agency.[19] This leads to costly delays in the recall process, which are especially important when a public health concern is present. PCA testing procedures had found salmonella present in their peanut butter 12 times since 2007, but the company was not required to share this information with the FDA or any state agency. Inspectors finally gained access to the positive test results by using a 2002 bioterrorism law against the company.

The sub-contracting of safety inspections by the FDA to state agencies has created uneven standards and enforcement procedures, under which companies are rewarded in the short term for manufacturing in states with loose food safety standards. The Georgia Department of Agriculture had even cut the budget of these state inspection teams, especially regarding the required travel to manufacturing facilities. Three samples from the facility were tested in 2007 by the state agency, while none were tested in 2006 or 2008.[20]

Corporate Responsibility

Along with improved government regulation, the long term safety of the domestic food will only be improved when better business and quality assurance practices are adopted all along the supply chain. The ability to trace the food throughout its journey from farm to fork is possibly the most important aspect of these improved business methods. This salmonella outbreak dramatically demonstrated the need for enhanced traceability because PCA's peanut butter paste was incorporated into numerous other products bearing the names of many other companies. Generally, the paste passed through several companies before the final product was received by the consumers, complicating the supply chain.[21] This supply chain integration is dangerous on both ends of the spectrum: it does not allow for informed consumer choices to be made because labeling does not clearly state where a product originated, and it slows the recall process because of the difficulty in retracing this multi-layered system.

Food producers, distributors and other industry members must also adapt their business models to consider improved quality assurance during production against the possible costs of loss of consumer trust and recall of products. PCA's failure to do this calculus led not only to it filing for bankruptcy but also a sharp downturn of sales for uncontaminated peanut butter products. Despite a hastily conducted marketing campaign by the rest of the peanut butter industry, sales of peanut butter fell nearly 25% in the aftermath of the recall.[22] A poll taken after the recall showed that U.S. consumers are becoming more cognizant of the existence of a recall, but not informed on the specifics. While a vast a majority knew of the recall and lacked overall faith in the food manufacturing process; a quarter of respondents in the poll mistakenly thought that major national brands had been included in the recall.[23] A preventative approach in valuation of quality assurance programs would have better served both PCA and the entire industry.

PCA could have been saved from this catastrophic recall by a responsive, diligent and ethical management team and more accountable employees. Documents obtained during the federal investigation of the facility show that products were shipped prior to being tested. When a laboratory official informed the plant manager of a positive salmonella test, he responded "uh-oh" and stated that the product was already on a truck going to Utah.[24] Many plant employees were poorly motivated to ensure product quality because they were paid only the minimum wage and had not received a raise in years. Management also informed employees when state inspections would be occurring and instructed them not to answer the questions of federal investigators during the recall.[25] To say the least, this type of management does not foster a healthy corporate value system or reward the type of diligent and ethical behavior that will be required to improve the food safety system. There will likely be criminal prosecution of certain PCA executives.

The regulatory structure currently in place to ensure food safety is outdated and inadequate to address our modern food production and distribution system. There has been positive discussion in Congress about empowering federal agencies to review food processing procedures, access company lab testing, and order mandatory recalls. In addition, more funding will be needed to allow federal agencies to hire more inspectors and develop better inspection methods. The new regulatory system should provide benefits for companies that show a commitment to food safety, such as quality measurement licenses that companies can place on product labeling. Conversely, companies that repeatedly violate the trust of the consumer by using inadequate safety precautions should be punished accordingly.

Ethical food company executives should welcome increased government regulation of the food supply chain in order to root out the irresponsible parties. Distributors of PCA products who were forced to recall their products should have been conducting proper oversight of PCA's operations and implementing an independent testing program. However, these distributors suffered greatly due to PCA's poor safety procedures, which could have been prevented by more effective government regulation. Additionally, companies and distributors whose products were not contaminated have lost a large amount of sales and profits due to the malfeasance of a member of their industry. Just like what occurred with recent spinach and tomato recalls, innocent farmers and small businesses have been the most impacted groups because of this peanut containing product recall due to their smaller profit margins and inability to weather an economic hit. All of these different groups within the food production supply chain would benefit from improved regulatory standards universally complied with or exceeded by every company.

Companies must strive for real transparency within their supply chain, which would allow for traceability of all ingredients going into a finished product. This would allow for more informed consumer choices, benefitting a company's long term goal of attracting and retaining customers. Additionally, tracing food would allow for more efficient recalls that would both take less time and could effectively target only contaminated products. Nurturing a set of ethical corporate values, including quality assurance and food safety protocols, is not just important for public relations, but is critical to restore consumer trust in the industry as a whole.

As set forth in this Manifesto, the average American also has a leading role to play in the improvement of food safety standards. As a consumer, individuals are able to effect change in business practices by purchasing products from companies that have shown a commitment to food safety and not rewarding companies that introduce food that is produced by cheap and dangerous processes. Citizens can actively engage in the political process to ensure that the most effective methods of food safety are implemented. The following exhibit will introduce the reader to the controversies and proposals affecting needed reform.

Exhibit B: Pending Reform

The nation's system for ensuring a safe food supply is in desperate need of reform. The antiquated priorities and regulatory structure are endangering many American's health in both the short and long term. As highlighted in this Manifesto, there are many problems that must be addressed by a comprehensive overhaul in order to secure the food supply and guarantee it into the future.

The problem of a food industry out of touch with its customers is not new in the history of this nation. As the food supply chain was industrialized during the late nineteenth century, many concerns arose that companies were not taking adequate safeguards to ensure food safety. The newly formed agricultural business interests managed to defuse the situation by using political influence, until the confluence of several events resulted in a crisis over American meat. Europe had banned American imports of meat due to safety concerns during the 1890s, which led to the introduction of some limited regulation. A few years later, a controversy arose when meat packers were accused of shipping adulterated meat to soldiers during the Spanish-American War. The coup de grace for the meat industry came in 1906 with the publication of *The Jungle* by Upton Sinclair, which described the horrendous and unsanitary conditions inside the Chicago stockyards. Sinclair actually wrote the book to expose the brutal working conditions endured by the immigrants in the stockyards. Instead the public was more outraged by the revelations of unsanitary conditions and their impact on food safety.

Later that year, President Theodore Roosevelt led the charge in the creation of the Pure Food and Drug Act of 1906. This law was the first attempt at regulating the food production industry on a national level by prohibiting commerce in adulterated food, establishing quality standards, and placing limitations on false advertising.

Today, we find ourselves in a similar position. Although regulation exists, the system of rules for the food industry have not been effectively updated or enforced. European leaders have begun calling attention to the possible danger of some American food imports due to safety concerns. Controversial recalls of adulterated products have severely damaged the credibility of the food production industry, and there has been increasing scholarly and literary attention to the problem of food safety. Again converging factors are pushing the federal government toward action and improvement of the quality of our food safety system.

While much disagreement about the details of such reform exists, there is a general consensus that something must be done to restore public trust that has been lost. The Obama Administration has created a Food Safety Working Group to advise it on improving the regulation of the industry, and Congressional leaders have proposed a number of bills to improve oversight. Many industry leaders are coming to the table to discuss these proposals because they have realized the cost of recalls in both dollars and public relations caused by bad actors within their industry. Activists and other consumer groups who have long championed such changes now see their opportunity to change the future food policy of the U.S. government.

Current Issues

There are many issues that must be addressed in order for effective, comprehensive reform to occur. The most visible of these problems is the current regulatory structure of the government agencies charged with protecting consumers. There are two essential problems that face the current agencies: a complex and ineffective structure, and underfunding of the FDA. The responsibility for regulating all food safety is divided between 12 federal agencies, which together use 35 different rule books to effectuate policy. This structure does not create accountability in a single entity. Additionally, the FDA, which provides safety rules for up to 80% of American food, has been consistently underfunded. Over the last twenty years, as other agencies have seen huge budget increases, the FDA has been forced to cut back on oversight and the number of federal inspectors.[26] Most recommendations for fixing this structure focus on the creation of one federal agency that is totally focused on the nation's food supply and has the power to enforce rules across broad sectors of the industry.

A related problem is the manner in which inspections of food processing facilities are conducted. In the 1970s, the FDA was able to inspect half of the food processing facilities in the country annually. During 2008, these inspections fell to only cover approximately 5% of domestic facilities, with even less inspection of foreign facilities. President Obama called this inspection ratio a "hazard to public health" and has promised to address this inspection system by providing more funding.[27] One government proposal is to increase the use of private sector companies to carry out these inspections. Use of such private auditors has been linked with conflict of interests because the company to be inspected is often paying inspector's fees and a lack of transparency because these auditors are not compelled to disclose their findings to any government agency. During the peanut recall, in early 2009, it was revealed that the private inspector that had certified the contaminated plant as safe did not even know that peanuts were prone to salmonella contamination.[28] An increased focus on private auditors would only be effective if better standards for certifying such auditors were created, and conflicts of interest were limited by making the upstream purchasers or retailers pay for the audits, not the suppliers undergoing the audits.

One of the biggest functional concerns that must be addressed by food safety reform is traceability. This element is crucial to the ability to view the entire supply chain in food production, which is critical in case of contaminated food and recalls. A bioterrorism law enacted in 2002 requires food makers, processors, and distributors to keep records of where their products were sold. However, during a recent investigation by the Department of Health and Human Services, 60% of the facilities surveyed were not compliant with this law. The survey also revealed that only 1 in 8 products could be traced back to where they originated. The companies involved in the survey blamed these shortcomings on difficulty in meeting the record keeping requirements, lack of knowledge about the requirements, and lax government regulation. The FDA also suffers from a lack of effective power to request records from companies before demonstrating that the food in question presents a serious health threat.[29] Reform efforts must focus on extending and enforcing these traceability requirements, as well as promoting new technologies that could decrease the cost of record keeping.

Globalization of food supply has created numerous, complex problems as the industry has sought to address consumer demand for exotic products and keep short term costs as low as possible. The United States imports an increasing percentage of its food, with $3.45 billion imported from China alone in 2008. Once food components are sourced from abroad and incorporated into highly processed food, they are very difficult to isolate or trace back to their source. The FDA's lack of resources means that only 1% of all food imports are inspected annually.[30] China has been the source of a number of high profile recalls and health concerns involving everything from medicine to pet food to infant formula. New laws were recently passed to reform food safety practices in China, but as stated below there will be huge implementation challenges. Yet, it is unfair to cast blame only on China. A review of the FDA Import Alerts listed on the FDA website shows that many other countries have been attempting to export adulterated and misbranded foods into the U.S. As a result, the FDA must have increased authority and funding to conduct border inspections, and the power to inspect all foreign food processing facilities seeking to export their products here.

Nutrition standards must be incorporated into this comprehensive reform to best promote the health of Americans. Many consumer groups have pointed to the fact that the food industry has become very good at producing cheap and abundant food, not necessarily healthy food. Government subsidies of food industries have tended to focus on this agri-business to the tune of $7.5 billion every year. Meanwhile, the organic food industry only receives about $15 million annually. The Obama Administration is already announcing new ideas to promote nutrition in school meals and vending machines, as well as increasing aid to locally grown health foods.[31] This focus on nutrition is important because it encourages consumer demand for healthier foods and improves the overall health of the American people.

As stated in the Manifesto, transparency must be legislated if the food industry as a whole will not voluntarily remove the burkas covering its quality assurance, food safety, traceability, animal welfare, and employment practices. Instead of just holding hearings where the bad actors are brought before Congress, our Representatives and Senators need to bring in the progressive companies (some of which are noted in the Manifesto) who are trying to lead the way with better practices.

Reform Legislation

At the end of 2007, the FDA announced a new food protection plan and requested expanded authority from Congress. These expansions would allow the FDA to establish preventive controls (especially for high risk foods), accredit private inspectors, charge reinspection fees for facilities failing the first inspection, increase inspection of imports, call for mandatory recalls, and access company records during food emergencies. There are numerous bills that have already been proposed in this 111th Congressional session to address the above problems and requests. Some of these proposals attempt to achieve comprehensive reform of the food safety system, while others only address more limited goals.

The bill receiving the most attention has been the Food Safety Modernization Act proposed by Rep. Rosa L. DeLauro (D-CT), who has long been a vocal critic of the food safety system. The main effect of this bill is to divide the FDA in two with an agency that regulates drugs and medical devices and another that focuses solely on food—the Food Safety Administration (FSA). This agency would be responsible for establishing a national food safety program that would control all aspects of food safety in the country. The purpose of this bill is to simplify the regulatory structure and create accountability in the Administrator of the agency. This bill deals comprehensively with the responsibilities of this new agency, including research and public education, and grants it enforcement powers.

The Safe Food Enforcement, Assessment, Standards, and Targeting Act (so called "Safe FEAST") sponsored by Rep. Jim Costa (D-CA) is another attempt at comprehensive reform but without dismantling the FDA structure. Rather than creating a new agency, the bill attempts to strengthen the current FDA powers relative to recalls, inspections, and safety standards for food companies. These powers would also allow the creation of a uniform standard for laboratory testing of food products, and improve regulatory capacity (safety practices, traceability, and surveillance). Imported food would require identification of suppliers and notice of food importation. The FDA would have the power to review foreign country regulation, inspect facilities within the exporting country, and provide the country assistance in improving its own food safety system.

The FDA Globalization Act sponsored by Rep. John Dingell (D-MI) is another attempt at systemic reform with many of the same features as the above proposals. Traceability would be addressed by establishing mandatory record keeping procedures for food producing companies. Mandatory recall power would be given to the FDA, as well as the power to access company records to effectuate this mandate. There is one controversial difference in this bill in that it would allow the FDA to establish user fees charged to food companies that fail one inspection, in order to help pay for subsequent regulation and inspections.

In the Senate, Dick Durbin (D-IL) has introduced the FDA Food Safety Modernization Act on a bi-partisan basis with Republican co-sponsors such as Lamar Alexander (R-TN). In addition to proposals aimed at the specific problems of traceability, imported food, and increased FDA regulatory powers, this bill would require all food facilities to adopt HACCP plans to prevent food adulteration and would provide the FDA with access to these plans. It provides guidelines and grants to schools to protect children with life threatening food allergies.

It is very likely that some measure of reform will be achieved because the political will is present more than ever before. Rep. DeLauro has commented on her optimism "that this could finally be the Congress in which we deal with this."[32]

Recent Developments

There have been a number of other developments in the food safety structure that could lead to an improved food security, supplementing the new regulatory system.

In the wake of the highly publicized recalls related to its food exports, the Chinese government is attempting to reform its regulatory structure. A new law was passed in February to create the National Food Safety Commission to coordinate between the five agencies that will retain daily supervision of the food production industry. The Commission will develop new rules that will provide guidance in every phase of food production, and it will create a National Emergency Plan to deal with adulterations in the future. However, a similar reform attempt in 2003 failed due to the crucial issue that still remains—scope. China's food production industry includes 200 million farmers and 500,000 food processing facilities.[33] There is no way the government can effectively monitor and inspect this many possible contamination sources without devoting many more resources to the problem.

Traceability will be positively affected as advancements make record keeping easier and drive administrative costs down. Texas Instruments, IBM, Microsoft, Motorola, and other companies are already hard at work developing advanced electronic tagging systems that are and will be even better able to trace foods from farm to fork. Much of this technology is already being used by logistics companies to track shipments.

Many small farmers have said that the cost of such systems would be prohibitive.[34] However, as demand for these systems rise and cost falls, this technology will become increasingly realistic across all segments of the food industry.

Many lessons can be learned about improving import regulation by looking to international examples. The European Union has taken the lead in most areas of food safety. Their system focuses on requiring countries wishing to import food to establish food safety standards roughly equivalent to their own, enforced by stringent border inspection procedures. In Japan, the inspection rate for imported food is more than 10 times higher than that of the U.S. Additionally, a special class of high risk food is even more heavily inspected. The Canadian system focuses on licensing programs for both governments and companies that wish to import food. Entities that repeatedly offend all of the above systems are subject to economic penalties and sanctions. These systems are not prohibited by any international trade agreements, which allow for domestic governments to enact laws "necessary to protect human, animal, or plant life or health."[35]

Exhibit C: School Lunches

There are 53 million young people in the public educational system in the United States that could be positively affected by better nutrition and safety standards for meals prepared in their schools.[36] Introducing healthy eating habits to school age children could help address the growing childhood obesity problems noted in the Manifesto and create a more informed future generation of consumers.

Ensuring the safety of the food supply is an additional concern because of the potential impact school food has on this already at risk group. During a typical school day up to 50% of a child's caloric intake comes from food provided at school, and a majority of all public schools have closed campuses restricting the child's food options.[37] These concerns have come under increasing public scrutiny with the rash of recent recalls contaminating the nation's school food supply involving beef and peanut butter.

Recently, a young mother, with a son attending a rural school in Arkansas, told me her son was served a peanut butter snack that had been recalled. The mom had been checking the peanut product recall list on the FDA website to make sure she did not purchase any recalled products for her family. She threw the snack away and alerted the school which apparently was unaware that the product had been recalled. After hearing about this incident, I inquired at school districts in three Arkansas towns (including the town I live in). All three districts subscribe to the FDA and USDA recall list serves which provide immediate email notification when food products are recalled. This is good news.

I asked relatives and friends (two of whom are teachers) to inquire with their local school districts in Illinois, Texas, Florida, and Maine about how the districts assure that recalled products are not served to the children. The five school districts contacted in these four states are urban, suburban and rural. This informal survey revealed that three of the five school districts subscribe to the FDA and USDA recall list serves. Two school districts surveyed were not aware that these free government subscription services exist. The latter districts rely on their food service vendors and serve whatever the vendors deliver. This process is certainly less timely and accurate than directly subscribing to the agency list serves. If a food service vendor fails to notify a school district about a recalled product, and the district itself is not subscribing to the FDA and USDA list serves, it is easy to see how a school could serve students food that is recalled after its delivery date.

My surveyors also sent me the school lunch menus their districts have developed for the children. All five of the school districts are serving whole grains, fruits and vegetables not just processed foods like hot dogs. Some of the lunch menus even provide the calorie intake for each meal – something that only a few restaurant chains do.

Healthy Food

Of course, improving the food choices of Americans begins with ensuring they have enough to eat and educating children on the benefits of healthy foods. The federal government officially began trying to address these needs in 1946 with the establishment of the National School Lunch Program to provide healthy, low cost meals to schools. Today, this program operates in over 101,000 schools, encompassing both the public and non-profit private sector. The program provides meals to over 30.5 million students every day by providing schools with cash subsidies and donations of food from the Department of Agriculture. Schools receiving these benefits must provide meals for students that meet the Dietary Guidelines for Americans, which are produced by the Department of Health and Human Services periodically.

In addition to assisting with nutritious meals, the National School Lunch Program also provides free or reduced cost lunches to children from low income families. Children coming from families below 130% of the poverty level are eligible for free lunches, while families below 185% of the poverty level qualify for reduced cost lunches. Local school food authorities establish the cost to be paid by other students that do not qualify for free or reduced cost lunches; however, to receive government assistance these programs must be operated on a not for profit basis.[38]

Due to the success of the lunch program, the federal government has added many supplemental food assistance programs. The School Breakfast Program mirrors the lunch system by providing subsidized meals for students and requiring schools to meet certain nutritional guidelines. A summer food program assists students of low income families during the summer break and other extended school holidays. Additional programs address the nutrition of after school snacks, the introduction of children to fruits and vegetables, and the provision of milk to students not participating in other programs.[39]

While the federal government does provide considerable funding for school meals, local authorities in conjunction with state agencies have discretion about the food to be served and how it will be prepared. The resulting situation is wide ranging disparities in food standards, and many criticisms of how these programs are administered.

Whiled the NSLP spent $9 billion in 2007, many experts have stated that three times as much money is actually required in order to effectively provide wholesome food for students. Much of the current funding does not go toward food purchase, but rather administrative costs of running cafeterias.[40] Additionally, food not prepared in the cafeteria is not governed by any nutritional standards. These "competitive" food sources are present in 73% of elementary schools and universally present in middle schools and high schools throughout the country. These competitors are most commonly foods that are low in nutritious value and can be purchased from a vending machine or school store.[41]

A GAO review of the effectiveness of school-based nutrition efforts concluded that schools were making progress but further improvement was necessary and attainable. A national survey concluded that education about healthy eating habits had a positive effect on students, but many schools were spending a very minimal amount of time on this type of education because of competing academic interests. Another barrier to improvement is the offering of alternative foods of low nutritional value during lunch periods. The study found that the most difficult problem faced by the school food authorities was finding a balance between the competing goals of nutrition, budgetary constraints, and providing foods that are appealing to students. The GAO report concluded that promotion of nutrition education and more effective state government collaboration with individual schools would most effectively address these challenges.[42]

While the federal government provides a baseline for state nutrition standards, many states have established more stringent nutritional requirements. The federal standards have not been updated in many years, and a recent study found that a majority of states were doing poorly in promoting nutrition in schools by themselves. Additionally, only 12 states had implemented comprehensive food and beverage standards that are applicable to the whole campus for the whole day.[43]

Many programs have been started on the local level by concerned parents and consumer groups to get more healthy food into schools. One of the most successful of these programs has been the National Farm to School Program, which, as a non-profit organization, is eligible to receive federal subsidies for providing food to school. This organization connects schools to local farms in order to provide fresh, locally grown food to students. This is a very complicated process for both the farmers and school administrators, but the effort has proved worthwhile because of the rising concerns of childhood obesity. The popularity of this program has soared over the last few years, and it currently operates over 2,000 programs in 39 different states.[44]

The proposed Child Nutrition Promotion and School Lunch Protection Act of 2009 would attempt to address concerns over the lack of a comprehensive standard. It would require the Department of Agriculture to establish scientific standards for all food served on campuses, including vending machines and school stores. The federal government would also be required to update the Dietary Guidelines for Americans, which would have significant impact on standards for federal food programs.

<u>Safe Food</u>

Recent studies have found that food safety in schools is lacking and could be dramatically improved on all levels. In 2004, Congress passed a law updating the safety requirements and inspections for schools, but there has been little effective implementation to assist state and local governments in enforcing these requirements. New legislation at the federal government would likely require states to put in place the most modern food safety practices. Websites and databases providing information about food safety practices and recalls of contaminated food should be updated and required for each school district, which would make implementation and standardization easier for different districts and states.[45]

The CDC has researched food safety and compiled a list of strategies that would improve food safety in schools. Some recommendations focus on state governments regulating school food more vigorously and increasing coordination with outside interest groups, parents, and non-governmental organizations. The other group of recommendations focuses on better food safety education for cooks, school nurses, and school health coordinators.[46]

Recently, the hopes for more funding to achieve these goals became more feasible with large budget increases proposed for both school food nutrition and safety. Schools will receive additional funding to upgrade and improve nutrition programs. Meanwhile, the Department of Agriculture and FDA will receive funds to prevent food borne illness outbreaks and increase inspections of cafeterias.[47]

As safe food has moved to the forefront of the pubic conscience generally, adolescent nutrition has become more relevant specifically. The recent peanut butter recall demonstrates that school supply chains are especially vulnerable to wide spread contaminations because of their reliance on a few large-scale suppliers. More effective regulation of these suppliers and incorporation of more locally grown, fresh foods will help address these concerns. The federal government must establish better standards for schools receiving taxpayer money. However, continual innovation on the state and local level is also needed to improve nutrition and food safety in schools.

Exhibit D: Bisphenol A

In the last few years, much media and government attention has focused on various chemicals leaching or potentially leaching into infant formula, beverages and food from containers such as water bottles, soft drink bottles, baby bottles, sports bottles, plastic tableware, and the internal linings of cans.

One of the controversial chemicals is Bisphenol A (BPA), which is widely used as a starter material for the production of polycarbonate plastics and synthetic epoxy resins used in beverage and food packaging. BPA was first synthesized in a lab in 1891 and was originally used as an artificial estrogen, although it proved to be of little commercial value. Use of BPA remained limited until the 1950s when it was used to manufacture hard polycarbonate plastics.

When the federal government began attempting to regulate industrial chemicals in 1976, BPA was examined and tested by the National Toxicology Program (NTP). This study concluded that BPA was generally not harmful in current doses and established a standard for its lowest adverse effect. In 1988, the Environmental Protection Agency (EPA) used this NTP study to set a safety standard for human exposure.

When the FDA began assessing BPA, it found that most canned infant formula on the market contained the substance because it had leached from metal can linings. A *Consumers Union* report later found that this leaching could also occur in baby bottles when the bottles were heated. In 1999, the FDA publicly declared BPA safe for use in food and beverage containers after a thorough evaluation. Continued research in some other countries was contradictory, especially with regard to low-dose exposure.

This was the regulatory background of BPA in 2003 when the National Institutes of Health (NIH) nominated it for further government evaluation relative to effects on reproduction and early fetal and child development. Sciences International was chosen as the contractor to gather research for this government project and to provide assistance in selecting the scientists to sit on the expert Advisory Panel. This panel would eventually find that BPA was safe in 2006, but the integrity of the process was questioned after it was revealed that Sciences International had BPA manufacturers as corporate clients. After a government investigation of the potential conflict of interests, Sciences International was fired as the contractor, but the work that it had already done was retained by the Advisory Panel. During this time the NIH had also funded a group of 38 independent scientists, known as the Chapel Hill Panel, to study BPA and come up with their own conclusions. In the summer of 2007, this group released its consensus stating that BPA presented a risk to human health at current exposure levels. However, the final Advisory Panel report disregarded this finding and rejected linking BPA to health problems, only expressing concern for impact on fetal exposure.

In early 2008, a congressional investigation was launched due to the rising concern about BPA's effect on the health of children. During the investigation, infant formula manufacturers told Congress that they either have no procedure for testing their products for BPA or conduct very limited testing. The FDA told Congress that the basis for the current agency position was two research studies that had been sponsored by a group representing BPA manufacturers. After an evaluation by the NTP showed "some concern" about BPA safety, Congress requested the FDA to reassess its safety standard. During this period, health officials in Canada declared the BPA a "dangerous substance," and many private sector manufacturers began to voluntarily cease using it for polycarbonate plastic baby bottles.[48]

In September 2008, the FDA's Science Board Subcommittee, chaired by University of Michigan professor Martin Philbert, was asked to review the previous assessment that BPA was safe in food packaging. During this review, it was revealed that a research facility founded by Philbert had been given a $5 million donation by an outspoken proponent of BPA just before being named chairman of the subcommittee. Philbert had failed to disclose the donation to the FDA as a potential conflict of interest during the selection process. Once the donation was discovered, an FDA official investigated and concluded that there had been no disqualifying misconduct because Philbert's salary was not being paid directly by the donation. Despite some congressional objections, Philbert remained chairman of the Subcommittee.[49] During the subsequent review process, some state governments began to take the initiative by asking baby bottle and infant formula manufacturers to stop using BPA. In the meantime, Health Canada determined that infant exposure to BPA is dangerous even at low levels.[50]

The Science Board subcommittee's report determined that the FDA had created a "false sense of security" when it only used two studies to formulate an opinion, despite the existence of other representative evidence. Additionally, the report found that the FDA risk assessment had failed to account for the cumulative effect of infant exposure to multiple products containing BPA. The change of Administrations after the release of this report has led to some delay in making any progress to formulate a new standard.[51]

Public Concerns

The two main sources of BPA ingestion are polycarbonate plastic beverage containers and metal food can linings which are both pervasive in the consumer product market. A recent CDC study revealed that 93% of Americans have BPA in their bloodstream at any given time, and it may remain in the body for a much longer period than previously thought. These results suggest that BPA may be entering the body from even more pervasive sources than originally believed, such as PVC water pipes used in homes.[52]

Consumers can become educated by learning what products contain BPA, which has become easier recently. Many plastic products are now marketed as *BPA Free*, especially reusable water bottles, because many businesses have seen the value of making these options available for consumer choice and not waiting around to be forced to remove BPA from their products. If plastic products are not marketed as *BPA Free*, consumers can still identify the products by examining the triangular recycling symbols which are usually located at the bottom of the products. The number 07 accompanied by the letters PC or O and the number 03 accompanied by the letters PVC may signify that the product is capable of leaching BPA. While such plastics may always be leaching

BPA, contact with hot liquids can exponentially increase the leaching process.

For metal can linings, consumers should assume they contain BPA. One exception is Eden Foods, a natural and organic food company in Michigan, which is using cans with non-BPA linings at this time, but not for all products.

The American Medical Association conducted the first large scale study of human subjects in 2008, showing a correlation between high BPA levels in the body and diabetes, cardiovascular disease, and liver abnormalities. A separate medical study at Yale found a relation between the chemical and a loss of brain function affecting memory and mood.[53] Previous studies had already concluded that the estrogen in BPA disrupted endocrine functions by increasing the sugar production in the body. These studies suggested a link between BPA and breast cancer, prostate cancer, heart disease, and diabetes. A review of 218 published reports which tested BPA on animals revealed that 86% of the studies found a negative impact on the health of the animal.

In 2007, the CDC stated that low income people were more exposed to BPA because of the low cost of canned foods associated with its use.[54] Generally, the research has caused the most concern for pregnant women and newborn children because of their lowered immunity and inability to quickly process the chemical.

While the federal government is still contemplating the regulation of BPA, local government and private actors have taken action. Suffolk County in New York became the first place in the U.S. to pass a ban on BPA use in baby bottles and children's sippy cups, establishing fines for retailers selling products in violation of the ban.[55] Several states are considering placing various limitations on use of BPA, mostly dealing with protection of children. Connecticut, Hawaii, Maryland, Minnesota, and New York all have put forward proposals to eliminate BPA from children's products. California has already considered a bill to completely phase out the chemical, which was narrowly defeated in a vote of the legislature. Maine has suggested requiring disclosure of the presence of any hazardous material in children's products. Massachusetts is considering legislation to replace BPA where feasible and fund research into finding a safer alternative.[56]

Canada banned baby bottles containing BPA in April of 2008, based on their review of 150 worldwide studies of health. The Health Minister stated that the ban was a reaction to the dangers posed to newborns and young infants.[57] Canada has continued to study the presence of BPA in consumer products and recently found that the chemical was present in a majority of soft drink containers as well.[58] The European Union (EU) set daily intake standards for BPA based on a risk assessment performed in 2006, and the EU has found little problem with use of the chemical within these limits. The European Food Safety Authority has found that humans, even babies, are able to metabolize BPA effectively, so long as this daily amount is not surpassed.[59] However, the concern over possible dangers of the chemical in Japan led manufacturers to switch to ethylene for canned food as a substitute for BPA.[60]

To add to the controversy and confusion over this chemical, in March 2009, Food Standards Australia and

New Zealand (FSANZ) announced the agency's conclusion that BPA is safe for food and beverage packaging.

There are valid industry concerns about requiring the immediate removal of BPA in metal can linings. The most important of which is that there has been very little progress in finding a suitable replacement for BPA across all food groups. The BPA linings are needed to prevent corrosion and weakening of cans overtime, especially from highly acidic foods. There is at least one company offering BPA free canned food but the company's product line is limited and does not encompass highly acidic foods.

The industry has taken different approaches to the continued use of BPA in the face of a growing public concern and confusion. Industry groups like the American Chemistry Council and the Grocery Manufacturers Association have long fought for the safety and continued use of BPA, especially in metal can linings. During the mounting public attention to the issue, industry associations have maintained that the weight of scientific research supports their position, and consumers should not worry about the safety of the food packaging industry. After Suffolk County passed its ban on BPA, the North

American Metal Packaging Alliance stated the effect of the ban would be to restrict consumer's access to certain baby foods and bottles.[61]

However, several major companies have announced the elimination of BPA in their plastic baby products in an attempt to address market concerns. Connecticut Attorney General Richard Blumenthal, along with other state attorney generals, had been pressing companies for this deal and after the recent publicity, the State of Connecticut entered into agreements with Avent, Disney First Years, Gerber, Dr. Brown, Playtex, and Evenflo to discontinue use of the chemical.[62] Major retailers (Toys 'R Us and Wal-Mart) have responded to the consumer concern over BPA by announcing a phase out of the chemical in baby bottles sold in their stores. Sunoco became the first manufacturer to admit unknown health concerns about BPA and require all customers purchasing this chemical to guarantee it would not be used for children's products.[63]

In the meantime, The Ban Poisonous Additives Act of 2009 would amend the Federal Food, Drug and Cosmetics Act to deem any food 'adulterated' if it was packaged in a BPA container. This bill, introduced in the Senate by Senator Diane Feinstein (D-CA) and in the House by Representative Edward Markey (D-MA), would immediately outlaw sale and manufacture of food and beverage containers with BPA. The BPA-Free Kids Act, sponsored by Senator Charles Schumer (D-NY), attempts to ban BPA for consumer products for use by or for the care of children under the age of seven. This bill would also allow states to enact greater measures of protection if they so desired and require more thorough study of the health effects of BPA, especially relating to pregnant women.[64]

However, perhaps the most desirable process for creating a solution for this issue, especially for metal can linings, where the industry concern over lack of current alternatives deserves recognition, is compromise. Instead of an immediate federal ban, perhaps a phased in elimination of BPA in metal can linings would be more reasonable to allow the development of viable substitutes. Frankly, the stakeholders (consumer advocacy groups and industry) on this issue could learn from the progress made between opposing groups in other areas of law at the state level. In Arkansas recently, years of conflict and impasse between animal welfare groups on one side and hunters and farmers on the other, was resolved by Attorney General Dustin McDaniel bringing the opposing sides together to negotiate a compromise bill. In February 2009, Arkansas Governor Mike Beebe signed into law new animal cruelty restrictions that make aggravated cruelty to cats, dogs and horses a felony on the first offense, without unreasonable infringements on the traditional agricultural and hunting way of life in the state. Groups that supported the new law include the Arkansas Game and Fish Commission, the Arkansas Farm Bureau, the Arkansas Poultry Federation, the Arkansas Prosecuting Attorneys Association, and The Humane Society of the United States.

If applied to the BPA controversy, this type of give and take could allow industry to express concerns about the immediate removal of BPA from metal cans and sufficient time to develop substitute linings that protect the integrity of cans while addressing health concerns.

This is a more effective way to solve problems unlike the process in Washington D.C., where massive amounts of money are spent on oppositional lobbying by both sides of issues; with the result that many important issues are stalemated for years (for example, immigration reform).

BPA is only one of several chemicals used in the packaging of food and consumer products, only to discover potentially harmful effects from its use later. Many of these chemicals were introduced to the manufacturing process during a time when thorough scientific evaluation was very difficult or impossible. Today, modern scientific advancements have made it possible for us to more accurately gauge the potential health risks of a chemical. However, this evaluation must occur in an honest, unbiased and transparent manner. Too often, government regulators and industry groups view their relationship as adversarial, and consumers are usually the victim of this relationship. There are some fringe consumer groups which exaggerate the health risks of a product to galvanize their membership.

THE ETHICAL FOOD MANIFESTO

Consumers must use their purchasing power to demand purely scientific evaluation of chemicals that will be incorporated into food and consumer products and reward those companies that demonstrate a commitment to precaution and safety.

Exhibit E: Supplements

Natural herbs have been used for centuries in Eastern medical practice both as cures for certain maladies and as supplements to maintain good health. In recent years, these types of treatments have seen resurgence as an alternative to modern pharmaceuticals, often in an attempt to treat problems that Western medicine cannot cure. This "alternative" medicine has provided relief for some people suffering a variety of ailments such as back pain, the common cold, and more serious ailments. However, one of the modern incarnations of this type of treatment has caused rising concerns for many doctors, scientists, and consumers.

Dietary supplements are sold in pill form by retailers across the country without the requirement of a prescription. These products promise an almost unlimited variety of health benefits including weight loss, increased mental acuity, and additional nutrition. The practice of diagnosing and treating one's own health problems has led to many questions about the ingredients contained in the pills, the source of these ingredients, and the veracity of claimed health benefits.

These questions have been exacerbated with the recent investigations of some companies and the recall of products, but answers have been difficult to ascertain due to the complexity of the modern supply chain and the lack of effective government oversight. Scientists and food safety experts worry about the effects of vitamins either as ineffective placebos or as a growing danger to public health. Consumers remain largely unaware of the possible problems with supplements, and industry is split between those who like their current profit margins and those who think the long term viability of the industry would be improved by better government regulation.

Industrialization of the food and drug supply chain led to the profusion of many new products on the market, accompanied by many new consumer concerns. Vitamins and supplements were already widely used in the United States when they were introduced in pill form during the 1930s. A rising concern for public safety led Congress to pass the Food, Drug, and Cosmetic Act of 1938, which gave the FDA power to regulate the contents and claims of products meant for human consumption. The agency divided its reviewing standard between foods—which included vitamins and supplements—and drugs—any substance that had a demonstrated effect on curing or treating disease. This system remained in place in the latter half of the twentieth century as many American consumers became increasingly concerned with nutrition and healthy lifestyles. In response to this consumer demand, many food and supplement companies began aggressive marketing campaigns claiming all sorts of intended health benefits. During the late 1980s the FDA began trying to regulate these claims and ensure their accuracy.[65] These events laid the ground for the modern political struggle over the regulation of dietary supplements.

The Nutrition Labeling Act, originally introduced by Rep. Henry Waxman (D-CA), was passed in 1990 to set the rules on what beneficial effects manufacturers could claim on packaging for food and drugs. This law drew the attention of Senator Orrin Hatch (R-UT) who personally used supplements and politically needed them. Hatch's home state of Utah is a nexus for the dietary supplement industry, which currently represents the state's third largest industry. Hatch has received numerous political contributions from the industry and has owned shares in a dietary supplement company. His political interests and personal background made him a champion for the dietary supplement industry and opponent of this new law that extended government oversight.

Waxman's new law required a Nutrition Box on every product disclosing its ingredients and required any claimed health benefit to be reviewed by the FDA to meet a standard of "significant scientific agreement." The FDA began formulating a wide variety of regulations to enforce this new law, and Waxman introduced another bill to give the agency the subpoena power it would require to enforce its new powers. In an attempt to delay these regulations from taking effect, Hatch (along with then Rep. Bill Richardson) proposed a one year moratorium on all new FDA regulations related to supplements. Simultaneously, the industry interests launched a public advertising campaign with celebrity endorsements and dire warnings of FDA raids on alternative medical facilities. These efforts led to the failure of Waxman's bill for FDA subpoena power, and President George H.W. Bush signing into law the year long delay in implementation of the FDA's new rules. After beating back the attempt at increased oversight, the industry began to look for more pro-active legislation that would keep the government from regulating supplements in the future.

Hatch proposed a bill that would amend regulations to make clear supplements were to be regulated as foods, not drugs, by the FDA. Although the bill retained the standard of "significant scientific agreement" for companies making health claims, it also allowed the much less stringent standards of "totality of scientific evidence" and "truthful and non-misleading." During the subsequent debate, the head of the FDA voiced concern that there were problems with some supplements that masquerade as drugs in disguise, and he warned that a product's risk does not diminish when marketed as a supplement rather than a drug. The industry again countered this testimony with an aggressive public opinion campaign that told consumers the federal government was trying to limit their free choice. This advertising campaign combined with many people's strong belief in the effectiveness of alternative medicine, to push public sentiment behind the Hatch bill. Eventually opponents could no longer delay the bill in congressional committees, and the Dietary Supplement Health and Education Act (DSHEA) was passed in October of 1994.[66]

Current Regulatory Framework

DSHEA, which amended the Food, Drug and Cosmetic Act of 1938, established the modern framework for regulation of dietary supplements. It expands the definition of a dietary supplement to include products intended for consumption in pill, tablet, or capsule form and containing any combination of a vitamin, mineral, herb, botanical substance, amino acid, metabolite, concentrate, constituent, extract, or other dietary supplement. The packaging of these products has to state it is being sold as a dietary supplement, rather than as conventional food. Inclusion of any "new ingredient," that was not being used in the United States prior to the passage of the Act, required the manufacturer to give reasonable evidence that the substance was safe for human consumption. Manufacturers of dietary supplements were required to register with the federal government, but they did not have to provide a list of their products on the market. Labels were to be placed on every product identifying the product's manufacturer and providing a list of ingredients. However, proprietary blends of ingredients were only required to list their ingredients by order of predominance, not actual content, because of their secretive nature.

The controversial issue of claimed health benefits was resolved by allowing manufacturers to make three types of claims that could pass the loose "totality of scientific evidence" standard. Health claims could be made based on an established relationship between the contents of the supplement and diseases or heart related conditions. Claims about nutrient content could be made based on the relative amount of substances present in a supplement. 'Structure-Function' claims could be made based on effect of the ingredients on organs and systems of the body but could not claim to cure or treat a disease. These final types of claims must be submitted to the FDA prior to market release and a disclaimer must state that the claims have not been approved by the FDA.[67] The Federal Trade Commission (FTC) regulates how these types of claims are made in product advertising and has been fairly active in bring suits against companies.

The FDA cannot conduct pre-market review of dietary supplements, and they are not required to be proven safe by the company. Safety monitoring consists of mandatory reporting by companies of any serious adverse event (death or hospitalization) related to their product; voluntary reporting of any adverse events by doctors and consumers; and agency review of product labeling and accompanying literature, as resources permit. The FDA may also take action against products marketed as a cure for specific diseases or alleviating disease symptoms.[68]

However, the FDA is just as constrained in enforcement of regulations as it is in reviewing products. In order to remove a product from the market the FDA must prove the product is dangerous, which is a cumbersome standard for the prevention of public health outbreaks. In 2006, a panel at the National Institutes of Health stated that FDA has insufficient resources and authority to require necessary information from the dietary supplement companies. The panel concluded that these constraints "make it difficult for the health of the American people to be adequately protected."[69]

Public Concerns

While a majority of supplement companies produce quality products, this regulatory atmosphere has allowed some bad actors to prosper and create serious public health problems. The entire business model of the industry must be changed to create more openness and honesty in product marketing, ingredient composition, ingredient importation, and pre-market product testing.

Despite the allowance of many types of beneficial claims to be made by supplement manufacturers, there has been a continuing problem of companies making unproven, misleading claims of beneficial effects. The basic requirement for all FTC regulation of advertising claims is that they must be truthful, not misleading, and be adequately substantiated. Substantiation of dietary supplement claims is based on a standard of "competent and reliable scientific evidence" relative to what an expert in the field would consider to be adequate. There are no set protocols for what will be sufficient evidence to make a valid claim, but there are specific limitations placed on expert endorsements and claims based on traditional use of the product. DSHEA does require that every product display a disclaimer stating that the FDA has not approved the product and that it cannot cure diseases.

Advertisements claiming to treat or to cure disease are particularly onerous because they can prey on desperate people and may interfere with other treatments. The FTC commonly brings claims against the companies for deceptively marketing herbal supplements as cures for a range of diseases.[70] Many companies use highly effective infomercials which drive hundreds of millions of dollars in sales. In 2005, one FTC Commissioner said that stations running misleading infomercials should be held liable for false advertising, but this recommendation has not yet been adopted.[71]

The rise of the internet makes monitoring all supplement advertising virtually impossible and increases availability for children. A report in the Journal of the American Medical Association stated that more than half of 400 internet sites surveyed were making illegal claims related to the sale of supplements. Adding to this problem, consumers are generally not informed about what can be legally claimed on a supplement packaging. In 2002, a nationwide poll showed that over half of the respondents mistakenly believed that supplements had to be approved by the federal government, warnings of side effects had to appear on labeling, and claims had to be established with rigorous scientific proof.[72]

Along with improper marketing procedures, the constituent ingredients of supplements may be related to some health problems. This is commonly due to ingredients that are undisclosed, unknown or mixed with prescription medication. Labels require all ingredients to be listed except in the case of proprietary blends because this would force the company to disclose a trade secret. These types of blends are only required to list their ingredients in their order of predominance in the product, meaning that the amount of a substance in a product is unknown in many instances.

Additionally, there have been many documented cases of a supplement either not containing a claimed ingredient or not disclosing some ingredient that is contained in the product. These examples were very high profile and should be familiar to most readers.

StarCaps was marketed as a natural weight loss supplement and was used by athletes and celebrities for many years. It was also among the dozens of weight loss supplements found to be containing undisclosed ingredients during a recent FDA investigation. StarCaps contained a pharmaceutical drug called bumetanide, which can prove toxic when mixed with other medications. When this contamination came to light the weakness in the supply chain became apparent. The retailer claimed reliance on the assurances of the manufacturer, and the manufacturer stated that she was "shocked" by the news before recalling the product. The manufacturer and retailer now face lawsuits by some consumers who had been using the StarCaps for weight loss—including the high profile case of professional football player who failed a drug test due the undisclosed ingredient.[73]

Actra-RX was marketed by Body Basics as a "natural sex enhancer," but tests showed that it contained a significant amount of the active ingredient used in the pharmaceutical Viagra. This ingredient was not disclosed on the labeling, which also did not warn of potential harmful side effects associated with lowering blood pressure that would have accompanied an approved drug. When the FDA approved Viagra it required a warning on the product not to use with nitrates due to this potential health risk associated with this active ingredient. The reason that this ingredient was not detected was that it was labeled as a "dietary supplement," rather than a pharmaceutical drug. This led the FDA to warn at risk men, including diabetics and those with high blood pressure, and block further imports of the product at the port of entry.[74] While the same active ingredient was present in both Actra-RX and Viagra, only the one marketed as a dietary supplement caused sweeping health concerns because of a lack of transparency in the regulation of the supplement industry.

One of the main causes of ingredients being undisclosed or otherwise dangerous is the practice of sourcing abroad in countries that have very few safeguards put in place to ensure quality. An increasing number of supplements and constituent parts of supplements are being imported into the United States. China now provides 90% of the vitamins marketed in this country. This is because some ingredients can only be grown naturally in that country. Most ingredients are sourced in China to save on production costs. While the Chinese government has made many important steps toward reform, serious problems remain. Numerous small sized manufacturers continue to produce contaminated products and export them. The current regulations in the United States do not require supplement retailers or manufacturers to provide country of origin labeling, so it is impossible for a consumer to trace where the product's ingredients originated.

Establishing traceability is crucial to the safety of the supplement supply chain and the efficiency of conducting any necessary recalls. However, my informal survey of several supplement makers, including website reviews and phone calls, revealed that none of the companies will publish or disclose their traceability systems. Even retailers described as specialty or health food stores were generally unable or unwilling to provide some of the most basic information about where their products originate.

Fake exports of pills from China have been the source of complaints all over the world from Europe to Asia, where ineffective anti-malaria medications have surely contributed to spreading of the disease.[75] Apart from fake exports which actually do no harm, there are many exports that contain undisclosed ingredients that can do harm to consumers.

There have been well documented problems with a variety of Chinese products over the past decade, and there are encouraging signs that this may be addressed by both the Chinese and U.S. governments. During a high level trade meeting in 2007, an agreement was reached to allow FDA inspectors to open offices within China, with the main goal of capacity building by training private inspectors in the country. However, progress at meetings such as this one have been limited due to charges by Chinese officials that the Americans sensationalize the quality control issues, causing damage to China's national image.[76]

Many supplements have been around for thousands of years, but many others are very new creations that have not been extensively tested or studied.

The lack of required testing before products are put on the market allows pills with unproven health effects into the market. The long term effects of these untested products are especially problematic because the explosion of new product creation translates into limited clinical testing of the effects of the product over a period of years. Consumers who are unaware of the substances that they put into their body are causing unintended consequences that may not be realized for many years. Additionally, it is unknown what effect many of these untested supplements will have when mixed with pharmaceutical grade medication. Due to consumer assumptions about the limited dangers of supplements, a toxic mix of the two is very possible.

During the recent steroid controversy in the sports world, it came to light that one drug, known as DHEA, that acts like a steroid after entering the body had been exempted from the government list of controlled steroids. This product, which is marketed to the public as an anti-aging dietary supplement, was banned for over the counter sales in 1985 but allowed back on the market after the regulatory shift ushered in with DSHEA. The aforementioned Senator Hatch insisted on the product being classified as a supplement, not a steroid, despite the fact that many related substances were included on the banned steroid list because they metabolize into testosterone in the body. Reports of side effects related to DHEA have been limited to some facial hair and acne (mostly in women), but there have been no large scale clinical trials to thoroughly test it. While industry representatives have touted its good safety record and relative weakness as a steroid, the science behind the substance and possible side effects remains uncertain.

The preceding issues reveal a lack of transparency within the production and sale of dietary supplements that makes it difficult for consumers to make informed, intelligent choices. Misleading advertising has been widely disseminated due to the expanding market for supplements and spread worldwide on the Internet. Meanwhile, labeling requirements are insufficient to enable a consumer to determine the ingredients in many products or the various stops along the supply chain in the manufacturing process. Finally, studies of many dietary supplements have been inconclusive at best, especially with respect to their long term health effects, efficacy and safety.

Legal Reforms

There are many efforts underway in both government and business to improve the transparency of the dietary supplement industry. The FDA finally established a set of Good Manufacturing Practices for supplements in 2007. These standards, which will be fully enforced by June 2010, attempt to assure consumers of the identity, purity, strength, and composition of dietary supplements. Manufacturers are required to build a comprehensive set of process controls in production, not merely end of the line testing, to ensure that supplements are consistent in composition. Enforcement powers of the FDA for violations of the practices resulting in adulterated supplements include allowing the agency to remove products from the market and prohibit their continued manufacture.[77]

Additionally, United States Pharmacopeia, a nongovernmental group, has worked with the FDA and industry groups to establish voluntary quality standards and testing procedures. Products from participating companies are tested by the group and can use a "USP Seal of Approval" on their products. This licensing program is still very limited because it is voluntary and expensive, and only a small number of manufacturers have enrolled in the licensing system. Industry is beginning to express a desire for more regulation because of the damage caused to their products by some manufacturers and suppliers. However, industry does not share the view of the American Medical Association which has expressed a desire to see the supplements regulated more like drugs than foods, which could make the industry much less profitable.[78] Obviously some compromise must be reached before effective reform of the supplement regulatory structure can be achieved.

The Government Accountability Office released a review of the FDA's oversight of dietary supplement industry in January of 2009. It concluded the FDA had taken some steps to improve oversight but provided a list of recommendations to improve the overall effectiveness of this oversight. It stated that the FDA should request authority to require companies to identify and register the products they manufacture and expand the reporting of adverse events. The report continued by saying that clarity could be increased, if the FDA established guidance standards for foods that were fortified with vitamins and methods for determining the safety of new ingredients. The report concluded by addressing the need for increasing public education, which would allow consumers to make more informed decisions.

Internationally, most developed countries have established standards that are much more stringent in the regulation of the supplements than the United States. In Canada, a licensing system requires companies to obtain a product license in order to market natural health products. Companies must provide detailed information about the product and evidence of safety for human consumption in order to receive a license number, which must be displayed on the product's labeling. Additionally, site licenses are required for all stages of the supply chain and are obtained by manufacturers, importers, packagers, and labelers by providing evidence of quality control procedures. Japan has a highly regulated system focusing on the health claims that products may make on their packaging. The government has a list of standardized, approved claims that can be made by any product containing certain vitamins and minerals with established health benefits. Any claim falling outside of this list that makes a claim for physiological effects must provide regulators with information related to identity of the manufacturer and product in support of the claim's truthfulness, safety of the product and evidence of quality control processes. The rules governing the World Trade Organization, which generally govern most global trade, have no limitations on the ability of consumers to have access to dietary supplements.[79]

Consumer Lessons

Under the current structure, the dietary supplement industry has not done very much to create public trust in its business practices or transparency the supply chain. The rise and fall of the supplement Ephedra, which was marketed for weight loss, is a case in point. Practitioners of traditional medicine had managed to use the substance for years in a safe and, many would say, effective manner. However, once it was used in a concentrated form to create a supplement, its dangers became apparent. Industry and the FDA fought for years over the safety of the substance, but the agency was restricted from taking decisive action on removing the product from the market. It was only after public attention was drawn by the over a hundred deaths caused by Ephedra, that the FDA was able to step in and remove the product from the shelves. The industry responded to this ban in a demoralizing way. Within weeks they began substituting other stimulants, like bitter orange and green tea extract, that scientists had already expressed health concerns about, similar to the early warnings about Ephedra.[80]

Consumers must realize that educating themselves about the ingredients and effects of pill form supplements is crucial before beginning any "alternative" or self-diagnosed treatment. This can be accomplished by researching the product on numerous government and public health websites or by consulting with a doctor. Consumers should always consider and disclose every other medication or supplement they are taking during this consultation.

When making purchases consumers should look for products that have been subjected to an independent licensing program. These programs help to ensure safety and quality, especially the program operated by the U.S. Pharmacopeia. Additionally, large manufacturers with an established reputation are more likely to have preventative process controls built into their production. However, a supplement bottle that bears a recognized name is by no means a guarantee that the product is safe.

A final important point to consider is that the average person can fulfill their dietary needs by consuming a balanced diet and following the United States Government's Guidelines for Dietary Requirements. Supplements have a role to play for those with special needs, such as pregnant women and the elderly; but health consequences of the decision to take a supplement should be fully explored before any regime is attempted.

Acknowledgements

All author royalties from sales of this book will be donated to 501 (C) 3 non-profit groups combating hunger and educating children about nutrition. For more information about this commitment, please go to www.amcips.org, click on the "Contact Us" link. We will reply to your inquiry.

This Manifesto could not have been written without the excellent research and writing assistance of Stephen H. Terry, a 2008 graduate of the University of Arkansas Law School and a lifelong Razorback fan. I am very grateful to my husband, Theodore M. Hoeller, Sr. who surveyed food companies and encouraged me to write this Manifesto. I want to thank my relatives and friends who contacted their local school districts about the districts' recall notification processes and lunch menus.

Thank you Angela Hoy, Todd Engel and the entire team at Booklocker for designing and publishing this book. You are a pleasure to work with and you provide excellent service to your authors.

Appendix I:

FOR FURTHER READING

BOYLAN, MICHEAL. *Basic Ethics*, Upper Saddle River, New Jersey: Prentice Hall, 2000.

EHRENREICH, BARBARA. *Nickel and Dimed: On (Not) Getting By in America*, New York: Metropolitan Books, 2001.

GILLIGAN, CAROL. *A Different Voice: Psychological Theory and Women's Development*, Cambridge, MA: Harvard University Press, 1982.

GRANDIN, TEMPLE AND JOHNSON, CATHERINE. *Animals Make Us Human: Creating the Best Life for Animals*, New York: Houghton Mifflin Harcourt, 2009.

HUCKABEE, MIKE. *Quit Digging Your Grave with a Knife and Fork: a 12-stop Program to End Bad Habits and Begin a Healthy Lifestyle*, New York: Center Street, 2005.

KINGSOLVER, BARBARA. *Animal, Vegetable, Miracle: A Year of Food Life*, New York: HarperCollins Publishers, 2007.

LOVIN, ROBIN. *Christian Ethics: An Essential Guide*, Nashville: Abingdon Press, 2000.

MASSON, JEFFREY. *The Face on Your Plate: The Truth About*

Food, New York: W.W. Norton & Co., 2009.

MCNAMEE, THOMAS. *Alice Waters and Chez Panisse: The Romantic, Impractical, Often Eccentric, Ultimately Brilliant Making of a Food Revolution*, New York: The Penguin Press, 2007.

PATEL, RAJ. *Stuffed and Starved: The Hidden Battle for the World Food System*, Hoboken, New Jersey: Melville House, 2008.

POLLAN, MICHAEL. *In Defense of Food: An Eater's Manifesto*, New York: The Penguin Press, 2008.

POLLAN, MICHAEL. *The Omnivore's Dilemma: A Natural History of Four Meals*, New York: The Penguin Press, 2007.

NESTLE, MARION. *What to Eat*, New York: North Point Press, 2006.

NESTLE, MARION. *Food Politics: How the Food Industry Influences Nutrition and Health*, Berkeley, University of California Press, 2002.

NODDINGS, NEL. *Caring: A Feminine Approach to Ethics and Moral Education*, Berkeley: University of California Press, 1984.

SCHAPIRO, MARK. *Exposed: The Toxic Chemistry of Everyday Products and What's at Stake for American Power*,

White River Junction, Vermont: Chelsea Green Publishing, 2007.

SCHLOSSER, ERIC. *Fast Food Nation: The Dark Side of the All-American Meal*, New York: Harper Perennial, 2002.

SINCLAIR, UPTON. *The Jungle*, Ann Arbor: Ann Arbor Media Group, LLC, 2006.

SINGER, PETER ed. *A Companion to Ethics*, Malden, Massachusetts: Blackwell Publishers Inc, 1991.

SINGER, PETER. *Animal Liberation,* New York: Random House, 1975.

End Notes

[1] Clauson, Annette. "Despite Higher Food Prices, Percent of U.S. Income Spent on Food Remains Constant" Amber Waves; September 2008.

[2] Meade, Birgit. "Food CPI, Prices and Expenditures: Expenditures on Food by Selected Countries, 2007," Table 97, http://www.ers.usda.gov/Briefing/CPIFoodAndExpenditures/Data/2007table97.htm

[3] See, www.us.bbb.org/advertisers4healthykids.

[4] Leonard Doyle, American Songbirds Are Being Wiped Out by Banned Pesticides, April 4, 2008 at http://www.commondreams.org/archive/2008/04/04/8093.

[5] See, Singer, Peter. "A Companion to Ethics," Malden, Massachusetts: Blackwell Publishers Inc. 1991; Boylan, Michael. "Basic Ethics": Upper Saddle River, New Jersey: Prentice Hall, 2000; and The Ayn Rand Institute (www.aynrand.org).

[6] The House of Representatives Energy and Commerce Committee's Subcommittee on Oversight and Investigations held a hearing titled, "The Salmonella Outbreak: The Role of Industry in Protecting the Nation's Food Supply" on March 19, 2009 in 2123 Rayburn House Office Building. This hearing examined the actions and obligations of manufacturers and

retailers that purchased tainted peanut products from the Peanut Corporation of America (PCA). Documents and video from the hearing are posted on the Committee's website at http://www.enegrycommerce.house.gov/index2.php?option=com_content&task=view&id=1541Itemid=95, accessed on April 4, 2009.

[7] Stone, Brad and Richtel, Matt. "Forging a Hot Link to the Farmer Who Grows the Food," *The New York Times*, March 28, 2009. http://www.nytimes.com/2009/03/28/technology/internet/28farmer.html?scp=1&sq=eater,%20meet%20your%20farmer,%20and%20say%20hello&st=cse.

[8] Peltier, Michael, "Crist first governor to meet with farm workers group since 1990s," *Naples Daily News*. http://www.naplesnews.com/news/2009/mar/25/crist-first-florida-governor-meet-farmworkers-grou/.

[9] Ibid.

[10] Martin, Andrew, "Peanut Plant Contends Audit Found It in Top Shape," *The New York Times*, February 4, 2009.http://www.nytimes.com/2009/02/05/business/05peanuts.html?scp=1&sq=peanut%20plant%20says%20audit%20declared&st=cse.

[11] News-leader.com, "ATV Ban is not Sensible: Ban on children's toy shouldn't also apply to ATVs and motorbikes," April 3, 2009, http://www.news-

leader.com/apps/pbcs.dll/article?AID=2009904030312.

[12] Burros, Maria. "Supermarket Chains Narrow Their Sights," *The New York Times*, August 6, 2008. http://www.nytimes.com/2008/08/06/dining/06local.html?scp =1&sq=narrow%20their%20supply%20chains&st=cse.

[13] Hartman, Brian, and Kate Barrett, "Timeline of the Salmonella Outbreak," ABC News, February 10, 2009.

[14] Layton, Lyndsey, "Peanut Executive Takes Fifth: Lawmaker's Question Firm's President," *The Washington Post*, February 12, 2009, page A02.

[15] Moss, Michael, "Peanut Case Shows Holes in Food Safety Net," *The New York Times*, February 9, 2009. http://www.nytimes.com/2009/02/09/us/09peanuts.html?scp =1&sq=peanut%20case%20shows%20holes%20in%20food%20 safety%20net&st=cse.

[16] Blaney, Betsy, "Nation's Peanut Growers Reeling from Outbreak," *Associated Press*, February 15, 2009. http://www.msnbc.msn.com/id/29212000/.

[17] Jalonic, Mary Clare, "Who's Minding Your Food? Surprise! It Depends," *Associated Press*, February 24, 2009. http://www.msnbc.msn.com/id/29364630/.

[18] Moss, Michael, "Peanut Case Shows Holes in Food Safety Net," *The New York Times*, February 9, 2009.

http://www.nytimes.com/2009/02/09/us/09peanuts.html?scp=1&sq=peanut%20case%20shows%20holes%20in%20food%20safety%20net&st=cse.

[19] Harris, Gardiner, "Peanut Product Recall Took Company Approval," *The New York Times*, February 3, 2009. http://www.nytimes.com/2009/02/03/health/policy/03peanut.html?scp=1&sq=product%20recall%20took%20company%20approval&st=cse.

[20] Moss, Michael, "Peanut Case Shows Holes in Food Safety Net," *The New York Times*, February 9, 2009. http://www.nytimes.com/2009/02/09/us/09peanuts.html?scp=1&sq=peanut%20case%20shows%20holes%20in%20food%20safety%20net&st=cse.

[21] Severson, Kim, "List of Tainted Peanut Butter Items Points to Complexity of Food Production," *The New York Times*, January 23, 2009. http://www.nytimes.com/2009/01/23/health/23scare.html?scp=1&sq=List%20of%20tainted%20peanut%20butter%20items%20points%20to%20complexity&st=cse.

[22] Martin, Andrew and Liz Robbins, "Fallout Widens as Buyers Shun Peanut Butter," *The New York Times*, February 7, 2009. http://www.nytimes.com/2009/02/07/business/07peanut.html?scp=1&sq=fallout%20widens%20as%20buyers%20shun%20peanut%20butter&st=cse.

[23] Stobbe, Mike, "Survey: Peanut Recall Known but

Misunderstood," *Associated Press*, February 13, 2009. http://abcnews.go.com/Health/wireStory?id=6871943.

[24] Harris, Gardiner, "Peanut Products Sent Out Before Tests," *The New York Times*, February 12, 2009. http://www.nytimes.com/2009/02/12/health/policy/12peanut.html?scp=1&sq=peanut%20products%20sent%20out%20before%20testing&st=cse.

[25] Moss, Michael, "Peanut Case Shows Holes in Food Safety Net," *The New York Times*, February 9, 2009. http://www.nytimes.com/2009/02/09/us/09peanuts.html?scp=1&sq=peanut%20case%20shows%20holes%20in%20food%20safety%20net&st=cse.

[26] Senator Durbin, Richard, "Food Safety Reform: How and Why, " March 4, 2008. http://thehill.com/op-eds/food-safety-reform-how-and-why-2008-03-04.html.

[27] Harris, Gardiner, "President Promises to Bolster Food Safety," *The New York Times*, March 14, 2009. http://www.nytimes.com/2009/03/15/us/politics/15address.html?scp=1&sq=president%20promises%20to%20bolster%20food%20safety&st=cse

[28] Alonzo-Zalidivar, Ricardo, "Food Industry Safety Inspections Challenged," *Associated* Press, March 19, 2009. http://www.msnbc.msn.com/id/29775206/.

[29] Zhang, Jane, "Lack of Adequate Records Limits FDA," *The*

Wall Street Journal, March 26, 2009.
http://online.wsj.com/article/SB123810975105652717.html.

[30] Barrionuevo, Alexei, "Globalization in Every Loaf," *The New York Times*, June 16, 2007.
http://www.nytimes.com/2007/06/16/business/worldbusiness/16food.html?scp=1&sq=globalization%20in%20every%20loaf&st=cse.

[31] Martin, Andrew, "Is a Food Revolution in Season?," *The New York Times*, March 22, 2009.
http://www.nytimes.com/2009/03/22/business/22food.html?scp=1&sq=is+a+food+revolution+in+season&st=nyt.

[32] Rampton, Roberta and Christopher Doering, "US Lawmaker Blasts China Food Safety," Reuters, March 18, 2009.
http://www.reuters.com/article/FoodandAgriculture09/idUSTRE52H4LF20090318.

[33] Dickinson, Steven M. "Food Fumble," *The Wall Street Journal*, March 3, 2009,
http://online.wsj.com/article/SB123601731642111527.html.

[34] Hodgson, Jessica, "IBM Develops Technology to Improve Food Safety," *The Wall Street Journal*, February 18, 2009.
http://online.wsj.com/article/SB123498787316215281.html.

[35] Ward, Bradford L. and Lisa W. Armstrong, "Food Safety Reform: What the FDA Can Learn From Other Major Importing Countries," *Association of Women in International Trade*, Fall

2007. http://www.wiit.org/news/Fall2007/Reform%20F07.htm.

[36] Centers for Disease Control, Division of Adolescent and School Health. Strategies for Establishing a State School Food Safety Program. http://www.gao.gov/new.items/d09250.pdf.

[37] National Alliance for Nutrition and Activity. Update National School Nutrition Standards: Cosponsor the Child Nutrition Promotion Act and School Lunch Protection Act. http://www.cspinet.org/new/pdf/nana_fact_sheet.pdf.

[38] Food and Nutrition Service at the United States Department of Agriculture. National School Lunch Program: Fact Sheet. http://www.fns.usda.gov/CND/Lunch/AboutLunch/NSLPFactSheet.pdf.

[39] Food and Nutrition Service at the United States Department of Agriculture. School Meal Programs. http://www.fns.usda.gov/cnd/.

[40] Waters, Alice and Katrina Heron, "No Lunch Left Behind," *The New York Times*, February 19, 2009. http://www.nytimes.com/2009/02/20/opinion/20waters.html?scp=1&sq=no%20lunch%20left%20behind&st=cse.

[41] Robert Wood Johnson Foundation. Improving Child Nutrition Policy: Insights from National USDA Study of School Food Environments. February 2009.

[42] "School Lunch Program: Efforts Needed to Improve Nutrition and Encourage Healthy Eating" United States Government Accounting Office. GAO-03-506, http://www.saferstates.com/2009/03/bpa-states.html

[43] Center for Science in the Public Interest. Two-Thirds of States Get Poor Grades on School Food Report Card. http://www.cspinet.org/new/200711281.html.

[44] MacDonald, G. Jeffrey, "Food Program Brings Together Schools, Farmers," *The New York Times*, March 24, 2008.

[45] Center for Science in the Public Interest. Making the Grade: An Analysis of Food Safety in School Cafeterias. http://www.cspinet.org/new/pdf/makingthegrade.pdf.

[46] . Center for Disease Control, Division of Adolescent and School Health. Strategies for Establishing a State School Food Safety Program. http://www.gao.gov/new.items/d09250.pdf.

[47] Zhang, Jane, "Financing Health-Care Reform," *The Wall Street Journal*, February 26, 2009. http://online.wsj.com/article/SB123566834450884603.html?mod=relevancy.

[48] Houlihan, Jane, Sonya Lunder, and Anila Jacob, "Timeline: BPA from Invention to Phase-Out," Environmental Working Group Research, April 2008.

[49] Rust, Susanne, "FDA Looks into Gift to Science Center,"

Milwaukee Journal Sentinel, October 15, 2008. http://www.jsonline.com/watchdog/watchdogreports/3098757 9.html.

[50] "Houlihan, Jane, Sonya Lunder, and Anila Jacob," Timeline: BPA from Invention to Phase-Out," Environmental Working Group Research, April 2008.

[51] Szabo, Liz, "FDA Ignored Evidence when Calling BPA Safe," *The USA Today*, October 29, 2008. http://www.usatoday.com/tech/science/2008-10-28-bpa-fda_N.htm

[52] Biello, David, "Like a Guest that Won't Leave, BPA Lingers in the Human Body," *Scientific American*, January 28, 2009. http://www.sciam.com/article.cfm?id=bpa-lingers-in-human-body.

[53] Walsh, Bryan, "Concerns About Chemicals in Plastics," *Time*, September 25, 2008. http://www.time.com/time/health/article/0,8599,1841441,00.html.

[54] Rentas, Khadijah, "To Ban or Not to Ban: Bisphenol-A in Food is OK with FDA but Not with Some Scientists," *Columbia Missourian*, January 9, 2009. http://www.columbiamissourian.com/stories/2009/01/09/to-ban-or-not-to-ban/.

[55] Eltman, Frank, "NY County Lawmakers Vote to Ban BPA from

Baby Bottles," *Associated Press*, March 4, 2009. http://www.topix.com/city/smithtown-ny/2009/03/ny-county-lawmakers-vote-to-ban-bpa-baby-bottles.

[56] Center for Health, Environment, and Justice. State Initiatives on Bisphenol A. http://www.chej.org/documents/StateBPAInitiatives.pdf

[57] Layton, Lyndsey and Christopher Lee, "Canada Bans BPA from Baby Bottles," *The Washington* Post, April 19, 2008, page A03.

[58] Tobin, Anne-Marie, "Chemical Bisphenol A Found in Most Pop and Energy Drinks in Canada," *The Canadian Press*, March 5, 2009. http://www.google.com/hostednews/canadianpress/article/ALeqM5gsRNDe8IZgr3AUwiwYIJ-mE0DUwg.

[59] European Food Safety Authority. EFSA Re-evaluates Safety of Bisphenol A and Sets Tolerable Daily Intake. http://www.efsa.europa.eu/EFSA/efsa_locale-1178620753812_1178620835386.htm.

[60] Rentas, Khadijah, "To Ban or Not to Ban: Bisphenol-A in Food is OK with FDA but Not with Some Scientists," *Columbia Missourian*, January 9, 2009. http://www.columbiamissourian.com/stories/2009/01/09/to-ban-or-not-to-ban/.

[61] Eltman, Frank, "NY County Lawmakers Vote to Ban BPA

from Baby Bottles," *Associated Press*, March 4, 2009. http://www.topix.com/city/smithtown-ny/2009/03/ny-county-lawmakers-vote-to-ban-bpa-baby-bottles.

[62] Kindall, James, "Suffolk's Ban on BPA Hailed in Some Quarters," *The New York* Times, March 13, 2009. http://www.nytimes.com/2009/03/15/nyregion/long-island/15cupsli.html?scp=6&sq=canada%20bans%20bpa%20from%20bottles&st=cse.

[63] Staff Report, "Legislation Targets Chemical Linked to Disease," *The USA Today*, March 16, 2009. http://blogs.usatoday.com/betterlife/2009/03/legislation-tar.html

[64] The Library of Congress at www.Thomas.gov

[65] *The Congressional Quarterly Researcher,* "Dietary Supplements: Is Tougher Regulation Needed to Protect Consumers," Vol. 14, No. 30, pages 709-732, September 3, 2004.

[66] Hurley, Dan. *Natural Causes: death, lies, and politics in America's vitamin and herbal supplement industry*, New York: Broadway Books, 2006.

[67] Office of Dietary Supplements at the National Institutes of Health. Dietary Supplements: Background Information. http://ods.od.nih.gov/factsheets/dietarysupplements.asp.

[68] Center for Food Safety and Applied Nutrition at the Food and Drug Administration. Overview of Dietary Supplements. http://www.foodsafety.gov/~dms/supplmnt.html.

[69] Body, Jane E. "Potential for Harm in Dietary Supplements," *The New York Times*, April 8, 2008.

[70] Federal Trade Commission. Dietary Supplements: An Advertising Guide for Industry. http://www.ftc.gov/bcp/edu/pubs/business/adv/bus09.shtm.

[71] Hurley, Dan. *Natural Causes: death, lies, and politics in America's vitamin and herbal supplement industry*, New York: Broadway Books, 2006.

[72] *The Congressional Quarterly Researcher*, "Dietary Supplements: Is Tougher Regulation Needed to Protect Consumers," Vol. 14, No. 30, pages 709-732, September 3, 2004.

[73] Singer, Natasha, "F.D.A. Finds 'Natural' Diet Pill Laced with Drugs," *The New York Times*, Feb. 9, 2009. http://www.nytimes.com/2009/02/10/business/10pills.html?scp=1&sq=fda%20finds%20natural%20diet%20pill%20laced%20with%20drugs&st=cse.

[74] Food and Drug Administration. FDA warns consumers about dangerous ingredients in "dietary supplements" for sexual enhancement. http://www.fda.gov/bbs/topics/news/2006/NEW01409.html.

[75] Johnson, Tim, "China has Cornered the Global Market for Vitamins," *McClatchy News*, June 3, 2007. http://www.mcclatchydc.com/world/story/16535.html.

[76] Weisman, Steven R. "China Agrees to Post US Safety Officials in Its Food Factories," *The New York Times*, Dec. 12, 2007. http://www.nytimes.com/2007/12/12/business/worldbusiness/12trade.html?scp=1&sq=china%20agrees%20to%20post%20us%20safety%20official%20in%20its%20food%20factories&st=cse.

[77] Center for Food Safety and Applied Nutrition at Food and Drug Administration. Dietary Supplement Current Good Manufacturing Practices of 2007. http://www.foodsafety.gov/~dms/dscgmps6.html.

[78] *The Congressional Quarterly Researcher*, "Dietary Supplements: Is Tougher Regulation Needed to Protect Consumers," Vol. 14, No. 30, pages 709-732, September 3, 2004.

[79] Dietary Supplements: FDA Should Take Further Action to Improve Oversight and Consumer Understanding. GAO-09-250, http://www.gao.gov/new.items/d09250.pdf.

[80] Jaroff, Leon, "Beyond Ephedra," *Time*, February 10, 2004. http://www.time.com/time/columnist/jaroff/article/0,9565,589533,00.html.

Printed in the United States
146368LV00002B/3/P